Nursing Research

Biomedical Library
Queen's University Belfast
Tel: 028 9097 2710
E-mail: BiomedicalLibrary@qub.ac.uk

For due dates and renewals:

QUB borrowers see 'MY ACCOUNT' at
http://library.qub.ac.uk/qcat
or go to the Library Home Page

HSC borrowers see 'MY ACCOUNT' at
www.honni.qub.ac.uk/qcat

This book must be returned not later
than its due date but may be recalled
earlier if in demand

Fines are imposed on overdue books

Nursing Research

THE APPLICATION OF QUALITATIVE APPROACHES
Second Edition

by

Janice M. Morse

Professor of Nursing and Behavioural Science
School of Nursing
Pennsylvania State University
USA

and

Peggy Anne Field

Professor Emeritus
Faculty of Nursing
University of Alberta
Canada

Text © Janice M. Morse and Peggy Anne Field 1996

First edition published in 1996 by Chapman & Hall (ISBN 0 412 60510 4)
Reprinted in 1998 by Stanley Thornes (Publishers) Ltd

Reprinted in 2002 by:
Nelson Thornes Ltd
Delta Place
27 Bath Road
CHELTENHAM
GL53 7TH
United Kingdom

06 / 10 9 8

A catalogue record for this book is available from the British Library

ISBN   978 0 7487 3501 3

Page make-up by WestKey Ltd.

Transferred to digital print on demand, 2006
Printed and bound by CPI Antony Rowe, Eastbourne

Contents

Preface

This is a drastically revised and expanded version of the 1985 text, *The Application of Qualitative Approaches to Nursing Research*, originally published by Croom Helm. It was translated into Finnish and published (as *Hoitottön kvalitatiivinen tutkimus*) by Kirjayhtymä. Aspen acquired publication rights in the USA and Chapman & Hall in the UK. This edition will be published by Chapman & Hall and, in the US, by Sage as *Qualitative Research Methods for Health Professionals*.

In the 10 years since the first edition of this book, qualitative methods have developed enormously. Grounded theory has been explicated, and now, it seems, there are at least three types of grounded theory — that described by Strauss and Corbin, that described by Glaser and dimensional analysis as described by Schatzman. Ethnography has become a potpourri of styles and many schools of phenomenology exist, each distinct and with its own set of assumptions and proponents. Most importantly, observational methods have improved enormously with the advances in video technology, and, for complex and relatively confined settings, analysis of videotapes appears to be the method of the future. And as we worked on this edition, we were astonished at the number and quality of completed qualitative studies. In 1985 we struggled to find published examples; today we are delighted to discover that we now have the privilege of choosing examples.

Overall, perhaps the most important change has been in the **acceptability** of qualitative methods. While in some disciplines, such as anthropology, qualitative methods have always been the norm, other disciplines have been dominated by quantitative methodologists. In quantitatively oriented disciplines or departments, qualitative researchers felt alone and stigmatized. While there still may be enclaves of quantitative researchers, the most significant change is that qualitative methods have gained legitimacy, are now fundable by grant agencies and publishable in many journals — in fact, journals that specialize in qualitative methods are becoming more common. Most graduate research programmes include a qualitative course. Most importantly, grant agencies are recognizing the role of qualitative research in research programmes, and are now specifically calling for proposals with a qualitative component in some form of triangulated design. Qualitative research has almost come of age.

With such a rapid emergence of methods, inevitably there are some difficulties. With the exponential growth of qualitative methodologies, there is some cross-fertilization of methods as first-time researchers, working alone, try to fathom **how to do qualitative research**. Sometimes they 'do' whatever 'feels best' without concern for the epistemological origins or the assumptions that underlie each of the methods they are blending, and they inevitably end up with a result that, at best, is less than it could have been if assumptions had not been violated and, at worst, is invalid. We recognize that, although the best way to learn qualitative methods is to work with a mentor, there are not enough mentors available and methodology books are the only source available to some researchers. But where to start?

We hope that this small book will serve as a guide for those who are beginning qualitative research and are not very sure where to begin. The book is intended as a brief introduction and as an overview of qualitative methods. While a book of this size cannot be comprehensive, at least it is a starting point. This book is also intended to be used as an introductory text for research methods classes at the undergraduate and graduate levels, and to give the student a 'taste' of qualitative methods to balance the usually heavy quantitative orientation of such courses and the required statistics courses that inevitably follow. To simplify library work, it is recommended that this volume be read with a companion book of readings: Morse, J.M. (1992), *Qualitative Health Research*, Sage, Newbury Park. Those who are interested in grounded theory, or who are writing a thesis or dissertation, may also find the following volumes helpful: Morse J.M. and Johnson, J. (1991) *The Illness Experience: Dimensions of Suffering*, Sage, Newbury Park; and Field, P.A. and Mark, P. (1994) *Uncertain Motherhood: Negotiating the Risks of the Childbearing Years*, Sage, Thousand Oaks. Both of these volumes give more detailed introductions to the qualitative method; chapters consisting of the Results sections of student theses, and final chapters synthesizing the findings.

We are grateful to our editors who have helped bring this book to fruition. We thank our team: Dr Maritza Cerdas, Rhonda Harris, Bob Morse and Anna Lombard. Catherine Walker of Chapman & Hall and Christine Smedley of Sage Publications were our in-house editors, and most of all we thank Susan Dolan, Pennsylvania, who worked hard to ensure that what we wrote made sense and was comma perfect.

Janice M. Morse
State College, Pennsylvania, USA
Peggy Anne Field
Edmonton, Alberta, Canada
November, 1994

About the authors

Janice M. Morse RN, BS, MS, MA, PhD (Nursing), PhD (Anthropology), FAAN

Dr Morse is Professor of Nursing and Behavioural Science at the School of Nursing, the Pennsylvania State University and an associate in the Department of Nursing Research at the Milton S. Hershey Medical Centre. She has previously held positions as Professor and National Health and Development Research Scholar at the Faculty of Nursing, University of Alberta, Edmonton, Canada. Her major interests are in the areas of clinical nursing research, where she uses anthropological research methods to explore the concept of comfort in a National Institutes of Health (NIH) funded project. She is the founding editor of *Qualitative Health Research*, an international, interdisciplinary journal published by Sage. She has published seven books and more than 100 articles on such topics as cultural response to pain, childbirth, infant feeding, menarche, patient falls and research methodology.

Peggy Anne Field RN, SCM, BScN, MN, PhD

Dr Field is Professor Emeritus, Faculty of Nursing, University of Alberta. She has published in the area of maternity nursing, infant colic, student socialization, decision making and qualitative research. She has conducted research on such diverse topics as skills validation for maternity nurses; patient satisfaction with nursing care; helping the grieving mother; evaluation of graduates and community nurses' perspectives of nursing. Her interests include education for maternity nursing; nurse-midwifery; care-giving behaviour of nurses and ethnography, and the major focus for her clinical expertise is maternal – newborn nursing. Dr Field has held a McCalla Research Professorship, a Killam Annual Professorship and a Rutherford Teaching Award at the University of Alberta.

The purpose of qualitative research

1

> Research is to see what everybody has seen and to think what nobody has thought.
>
> (Albert Szent-Gyorgy)

Research fills a vital and important role in society: it is the means by which discoveries are made, ideas are confirmed or refuted, events controlled or predicted and theory developed or refined. All of these functions contribute to the development of knowledge. However, no single research approach fulfills all of these functions, and the contribution of qualitative research is both vital and unique to the goals of research in general. Qualitative research enables us to make sense of reality, to describe and explain the social world and to develop explanatory models and theories. It is the primary means by which the theoretical foundations of social sciences may be constructed or re examined.

Doing qualitative research requires the researcher to be methodologically versatile, to have an extensive knowledge of social science theory, to interact skilfully with others, and to be persistent, focused and single-mindedly committed to research. It requires that the researcher constantly distinguish between another's world and one's own, yet become close enough to the lives of another that it be both experienced and analysed. It requires that the researcher be able to conceptualize, to write and to communicate. Doing qualitative research is an intense experience. It enriches one's life; it captures one's soul and intellect.

Qualitative researchers begin data collection by examining observations and reports of the phenomena as they occur in everyday life. These data are then organized so that they are drawn together into a cohesive whole. Thus, qualitative researchers are primarily concerned with the development of description of an observed phenomenon to generate solid theory as an outcome, or the product of their research. As this theory is construed systematically, and even 'tested' or verified during the process of construction, qualitatively derived theory has minimal risk of invalidity.

On the other hand, in quantitative research pertinent knowledge from previous research and from everyday life is organized into theory — given what is known and one's best guess about reality — to build a cogent and best argument that may answer the question. This framework is then tentatively constructed as conjecture(s), systematically tested and subsequently revised in light of these experimental results. Qualitative researchers begin by exploring previous research, but instead of using it *carte blanche* as a framework, they tend to regard it suspiciously and place it aside. Rather than constructing a theoretical framework from which to work deductively, they tend to hold other researchers' work 'in abeyance'.

It is important to note that both qualitative and quantitative researchers are concerned with the construction of **solid** theory as an outcome. They put their energies into systematically developing theory, but their approach to this task is slightly different. The qualitative researcher's emphasis is on the **construction** of the theory, and the quantitative researcher's emphasis is on the **testing** of the theory.

The difference in approach may, in part, be due to the differences in the phenomena studied, the question asked and the techniques considered appropriate for confirming or refuting the conjecture. Quantitative researchers usually study concrete phenomena that have been examined to the point that they can be measured. The theoretical frameworks from which their hypotheses are derived are based on research that has been investigated and is not inferential. These researchers have some prior knowledge from which to work and a means to measure variables that are representative of the phenomena. In other words, they are able to propose a series of experiments that are reasonably 'low risk' and planned to incrementally **test** their theory.

On the other hand, qualitative research is usually conducted to explore problems about which relatively little is known. Qualitative researchers often cannot find adequate information to begin to formulate a theory about the phenomena. Often there is nothing from which to create a theory and therefore nothing to test. In fact, creating and testing a theory at this stage may be so far removed from reality that the exercise would be one of futility, frustration and luck; it would be inefficient and often absurd. Later in the chapter, indicators for selecting a method (quantitative or qualitative) and how the researcher selects **which** qualitative method is most appropriate, given known characteristics of a situation and the nature of the research question, will be discussed.

Each of the qualitative and quantitative paradigms has its own set of assumptions, established methodologies and set of experts. Because both qualitative and quantitative techniques are frequently associated with particular disciplines or linked to knowledge domains, there has, over the past few decades, been somewhat of a rift between the proponents of the two paradigms. Since the development of computers and the increasing sophistication of statistical methods, quantitative research has been more 'mainstream'. Quantitative research has been the normative mode of inquiry taught in universities, and quantitative researchers have tended to dominate review panels of funding agencies and the editorial boards of prestigious research journals. Because quantitative research was more common and considered the gold standard for research, qualitative researchers felt excluded, undervalued, and misunderstood. As a consequence, a **qualitative versus quantitative** debate of competing paradigms tended to be vented in the literature (Duffy, 1985; Goodwin and Goodwin, 1984; Smith, 1983; Smith and Heshusius, 1986). Fortunately, since the early 1990s , both 'sides' have come to appreciate the role of the other in developing knowledge, and a new trend of combining qualitative and quantitative research has emerged. Nevertheless, it is important to remember that both qualitative and quantitative methods are merely **tools** for solving research problems. It is the responsibility of the researcher to be **wise** enough to be able to recognize when appropriate qualitative or quantitative methods should be used, and **smart** enough to be able to do it. Such versatility is the hallmark of a good researcher.

From the perspective of considering research methods as tools, the qualitative — quantitative debate becomes an insignificant argument. The quantitative researcher's denigration of qualitative methods reflects a shameful ignorance of the role and contribution of qualitative research, and the qualitative researcher's resentment of the perceived quantitative researcher's control of research resources reflects the qualitative researcher's lack of appreciation of the common goal of the research process. Smart researchers are adept at both qualitative and quantitative methods, and they use the appropriate method at the appropriate time, according to the type of research question, the goal of the research and other considerations.

THE ROLE OF THEORY

What is it that we mean by a 'theory'? Theory is a systematic explanation of an event in which constructs and concepts are identified and relationships are proposed or predictions made. Basically, a theory is a hunch, a guess, a speculation or an idea that may explain reality. Theories guide investigation both in qualitative and quantitative research, but generally provide guidance at a different stage in the research process. In qualitative, inductive research, the researcher examines the data for patterns and relationships, and then develops and tests hypotheses to generate theory or uses developed theories to explain the data. Quantitative researchers, on the other hand, work deductively by testing developed theory.

Where, then, does theory come from? Given that theory is not established fact, but rather the researcher's 'best guess' based on previous research, others' beliefs, values and personal values, then theory is a framework, a perception of reality to be tested by research. Once it is tested and becomes 'fact', it is no longer a theory but moves into the domain of knowledge or 'truth'. Theory becomes more and more believable as it is tested and retested. However, the most important point is that theory, whether obtained inductively or deductively, remains conjecture, but, as it is tested, it becomes better confirmed. As they are derived from the researcher's present knowledge base and personal reality, theories are usually tied to paradigms associated with specific disciplines. Therefore theories are usually in agreement, rather than disagreement, with current trends. This aspect of research has received criticism (Feyerabend, 1978) because researchers tend to create and test hypotheses that for personal, practical reasons, such as ease of publication, will be consistent with established theories. They are more likely to select hypotheses that will be supported and will be statistically significant than to disagree with current thinking and risk statistical insignificance. Extensive and important theories, therefore, may continue to be used for prolonged periods of time (and sometimes even be supported by research), yet in essence be totally and completely wrong.

These 'errors' are most evident historically. The intense debate in the 1930s about the relationship between race and IQ (Brace, Gamble and Bond, 1971) or about the 'diseases' perceived to be caused by masturbation in the late nineteenth century (Engelhardt, 1978/1992) are excellent examples of how current values shape theory which was supported, albeit invalidly, by research. Unfortunately, as will be discussed later in this chapter, this trap for researchers and theoreticians continues today. Theory, derived inductively because it is derived from reality, is unlikely to be a product of the researcher's perceived reality or a distortion of the 'truth', although present-day values or personal biases are always a threat to validity. Nevertheless, theories are essential to the process of inquiry. As they are proposed, modified or refuted, they are subsequently replaced with stronger and more significant theories. In this way knowledge advances.

However, the theory has other important functions in knowledge development. Burton (1974) succinctly describes seven functions of theory in the development of knowledge. First, theory builds tensions within a discipline. It initiates dialogue and two competing theories may stimulate debate. For example competing theories of cancer causation pertain to stress, environmental contamination and genetics (Tesch, 1981). At the same time, however, theory stabilizes knowledge; for a theoretical explanation must, through publication, remain reasonably constant — stable enough to be tested, supported, modified, or refuted. Second, theory is 'counter-nihilism'. Theories develop to fill gaps in knowledge and to 'combat intellectual nothingness'. The third function is considering theory as 'temporality', for it places phenomena in time, anchoring observations in relation to nature and history. Fourth, theory clarifies by providing explanations for otherwise seemingly unrelated facts, selectively including, excluding or ignoring facts in the most effective and parsimonious configuration.

The fifth function is that of prediction. While a theory itself may fill a role of predicting events and outcomes, theory also serves to guide investigation one way or another, thus providing investigators with a systematic progression within a research programme, and preventing stagnation or random and haphazard procedures for research endeavours. Sixth, theory provides a means to 'show', reveal or disclose, drawing attention to particular phenomena simply because a theory **exists**, thereby drawing attention to a phenomenon. Conversely, the final function is that theory may also silence an area, by ignoring phenomena. Burton (1974) notes that this function may be essential, as some phenomena may require periods of social 'incubation' before they are examined by the scientific community. Thus, these seven functions, in addition to providing explanation, reveal that theory serves an important, almost political, role for science and society.

LEVELS OF THEORY

Theory has been classified according to its degree of explanatory powers — for instance one common distinction is that between grand theory and mid-range theory (Pelto and Pelto, 1978, p. 251). Grand theory attempts to explain a broad generalized phenomenon. As a consequence, the constructs tend to be abstract but the power of explanation is increased. Mid-range theory entails the use of more specific constructs, is more limited and is of lower order. Thus, the power of explanation derived from mid-range theory is more focused than in grand theory. For the purpose of this book, the focus will be on levels of theory that are addressed by the research questions selected and approaches used by the qualitative researcher, which are primarily mid-range theory developed inductively from low-order propositions and hypotheses.

In a professional discipline, research must eventually produce knowledge in a form that can be used to improve the practice of that profession. Theory forms the basis of knowledge development as critical concepts and constructs are identified and relationships between them demonstrated. Theory may be descriptive, prescriptive or predictive in nature.

TYPES OF THEORY

The goal of qualitative research is to develop theory using rich description, data synthesis and abstraction. Qualitative inquiry is a process of documentation, description, identification of patterns and concepts, identifying the relationship between concepts and creating theoretical explanations that explain reality.

However, all qualitative research may not have developing theory as the end product. For example the purpose of phenomenology is to identify the essence of an experience, and this is to provide rich and insightful reflections with which the reader may identify. On the other hand, the end product of grounded theory is to develop mid-range theory, describing a **process**. Note that the **product** of qualitative research is the theory. Qualitative researchers do not usually **test** a priori conceptual frameworks, but rather inductively develop strong and resilient theory.

Deductive theory

Deduction means to infer from what has preceded; in research, one therefore draws from previous knowledge in order to deduce potential relationships. Reasoning is the facility of deducing unknown truths from principles that are already known, and it is on this premise of logical inference that the scientific paradigm for research has been built. As deductive theory builds on previous knowledge and research, it is less likely to 'disturb' the prevailing paradigm unless competing tensions become strong. The work of Klaus and Kennel (1976) on bonding was adopted in the 1970s to provide the conceptual framework for considerable further research. Subsequent research assumed the correctness of Klaus and Kennel's findings, and hypotheses were generated based on their studies. However, research a decade later questions the findings of Klaus and Kennel (Elliott, 1983; Scheper-Hughes, 1992).

In most deductive research, hypotheses are generated from the researcher's knowledge extending from previous research, from library research and the results of others' work and from intuitive knowledge of the phenomena. This information is used to generate hypotheses by demonstrating relationships and testing the predictive value of specific variables. The problem is that when one is dealing with human behaviour, if it is studied out of context (such as in a laboratory), the context stripping that occurs removes many of the related variables. Thus, generalizations from findings may not apply outside the experimental situation. An excellent example of this is provided by pain research. Many findings of studies conducted in the laboratory have not been confirmed in the clinical setting (Chapman, 1976).

Deductive theory is most valuable when the researcher has clearly identified constructs and concepts with which to work. This situation is most likely when the relationships to be tested have been previously demonstrated, and there has already been considerable research conducted in the area. For example in physiological research these principles frequently hold true, but this is less often the case in behavioural research where the data are more subjective.

In deductive theory, the starting point is a set of concepts or a conceptual scheme. Some of the concepts will be descriptive, serving to show what the theory is about (health, hope, support and so forth). Concepts may also be perceived operatively, such as the degree of hope or the strength of support. The theory will then consist of a set of propositions, each stating a relationship and the direction of influence between at least two of the properties, such as the 'degree of hope varies with the strength of the support system'. Deduction also provides grounds for prediction or prescription. As theory is not fact (Morse, 1992), it is always subject to revision and modification.

Inductive theory

Inductive theory is directed towards bringing knowledge into view. It is generally descriptive, naming phenomena and positing relationships. It is frequently conducted in the naturalistic setting, and considers **context** as a part of the phenomena. The goal of the researcher is to identify patterns or commonalties by inference from examination of specific instances or events. During analysis the researcher moves from specific instances or data to more abstract generalizations extending from the synthesis of data, eventually resulting in the identification of concepts and theory development. Thus, analytic induction is an essential mode of inquiry by identifying variables in order to generate theory. When examining phenomena, concepts are defined and tentative causes and relationships are hypothesized. In practice, the researcher alternates back and forth between cause and definition, and, as understanding increases, the definitions, hypotheses and developing theory are modified.

The sequential use of induction and deduction

Grounded theory is: 'the discovery of theory from data systematically obtained from social research' (Glaser and Strauss, 1967, p. 2). Grounded theory is one approach in which the research is inductively driven, although both induction and deduction are used to develop the theory. Glaser and Strauss argue that if one conceptualizes from the data, and if data have been accurately recorded, then categories must arise fitting these data. Theory grounded in reality must provide an explanation of events **as they occur** and thus is less likely to be contaminated by prevailing theory. Because grounded theory explores reality as it occurs, it is concerned with **process**, and provides techniques that enable phenomena that change over time to be diagrammed (Corbin, 1986; Strauss and Corbin, 1990).

At the time that grounded theory developed, it was observed that social research focused mainly on the verification of theory, with the theory being modified according to the results of the testing. It was further argued that there was a prior step that was being neglected: the discovery of concepts and hypotheses relevant to the area being researched. The focus on verification as a technique for revising theory was a serious concern as the generation of theory necessarily precedes theory testing. As theory is linked to the data and provisionally verified in the process of theory development, it is, therefore, more likely to be valid. Grounded theory was a methodological approach that corrected this limitation.

EVALUATING THEORY

Theories are usually evaluated in research according to six characteristics: explanatory power (extensiveness of explanation), parsimony, empirical validity, internal consistency, usefulness and testing. However, in qualitative research some of these characteristics are less important, and another quality, the degrees of **fit** with the data (Glaser, 1978) is considered an important indicator of validity.

    Extensiveness is the ability of the theory to encompass the largest number of observations. As stated, 'grand' theories incorporate a larger number of observations than mid-range theories, and therefore have more importance and more significance than mid-range theories and models. **Parsimony** refers to the structure of the theory. If a theory is parsimonious, it consists of the smallest possible number of propositions, assumptions, and inferences, and is elegantly constructed. Next, **empirical validity** refers to the ability of the theory to 'bind' observations and data together and to give them meaning; and **fit** is the ability of the theory to provide a plausible explanation, one that is valid and true to the data. **Internal consistency** refers to the ability of the theory to be consistent in explanation about these data, without negation. It refers to the logical structure of the theory and its relevance to allied theories. This aspect, together with 'fit,' enables the evaluation of theory for **usefulness**. Finally, a good theory should be **testable**. Although testing theory is normally outside the realm of qualitative inquiry, qualitative theorists play an important role in theory construction, and, if qualitative research is to fulfil one of its important functions, these theories should be significant enough and polished enough for subsequent quantitative testing.

QUALITATIVE RESEARCH

In the previous sections, it has been suggested that qualitative methods should be used when there is little known about a phenomenon, when the investigator suspects that the present knowledge or theories may be biased or when the research question pertains to understanding or describing a particular phenomenon or event about which little is known. Qualitative methods are particularly useful when describing a phenomenon from the emic perspective, that is the perspective of the problem from the 'native's point of view' (Vidich and Lyman, 1994). In clinical research the emic perspective may be the perspective of the patient, caregiver or relatives. Qualitative research is usually conducted in a naturalistic setting, so the context in which the phenomenon occurs is considered to be a part of the phenomenon itself (Hinds, Chaves and Cypess, 1992). Thus, no attempt is made by the researcher to place experimental controls upon the phenomenon being studied or to control the 'extraneous' variables, all aspects of the problem are explored and the intervening variables arising from the context are considered a part of the problem. Using this approach the underlying assumptions and attitudes are examined, and the rationale for these are also elicited within the context in which they occur.

As previously mentioned, the qualitative approach to understanding, explaining and developing theory is inductive. This means that hypotheses and theories emerge from the data set while the data collection is in progress and after data analysis has commenced. The researcher examines the data for descriptions, patterns, and hypothesized relationships between phenomena, then returns to the setting to collect data to test the hypotheses. Thus, the research is a **process** that builds theory inductively over a period of time, step by step. The theory fits the research setting and is relevant for that point in time only. These data may largely consist of transcriptions of interviews, observations of the setting and of the actors. Data of these kinds are meaningful to others and considered 'rich' and 'deep' (Geertz, 1973). However, these data are hard to manage for the purposes of analysing and writing a report, as they cannot be readily transformed into numeric codes for statistical manipulation. In this respect they are often said to be 'soft' data.

The qualitative research process can be exceedingly time-consuming, both for the collection and the analysis of data. In contrast to quantitative research, the number of subjects in the study is necessarily small, and a random sample is not selected. Rather, the researcher selects participants who are willing to talk and have established relationships of trust with the researcher, or who are in key positions and have a special knowledge of the phenomena for one reason or another.

QUANTITATIVE RESEARCH

Quantitative research, in contrast to qualitative research, seeks causes and facts from the etic or 'world view' perspective (Vidich and Lyman, 1994). In this case the findings are based on the researcher's interpretations of the observed phenomena, rather than on the subjects' interpretations of events. Quantitative research looks for relationships between variables so that causality may be explained and accurate prediction becomes possible. The aim is to examine the experimental variables, while controlling the intervening variables that arise from the context. With this control over the effects of context, the relationships between variables will be generalizable and predictive in all settings, at all times.

Quantitative researchers establish a theory identifying all constructs, concepts and hypotheses while preparing the proposal and before beginning data collection. These concepts are made operational so that the hypotheses may be tested. Concerned with rigour and replication, the researcher ensures that the measurement instruments are reliable and valid. Data are then collected, numerically categorized, and the relationships between the variables used to measure the concepts are established statistically using 'hard' (i.e. numeral) data. Bias is controlled by randomly selecting a large and representative sample from the total population. Structured instruments, such as rating scales, are frequently used to collect data and are usually administered once, as it is assumed that reality is **stable** (the variables measured will not change over time). The techniques for research design and analysis are prescribed a priori in the research proposal, and there are acceptable, tested and appropriate written steps or guidelines to assist the researcher throughout the process. The goal of quantitative research is to test the theory deductively by systematically testing the hypotheses.

SELECTING AN APPROACH

In summary, the researcher should selectively and appropriately choose a research approach according to the nature of the problem and what is known about the phenomenon to be studied. Importantly, the choice of method depends on a number of factors, such as the nature of the phenomenon to be studied, the maturity of the concept, constraints of the setting and the researcher's ability and agenda.

Nature of the phenomenon to be described

The type of variables or the nature of the question may indicate that either qualitative or quantitative methods would be more appropriate. For example the purpose of the proposed study may be to examine the fears and anxieties of preoperative patients . Fear and anxiety can, to a considerable extent, be measured reliably and validly, quantitatively, using standardized anxiety scales. Physiological measurements of stress may also be used, such as hormone levels. Fear and anxiety may also be studied qualitatively by asking patients to describe their fears and feelings about impending surgery.

Consider the purpose of the study. Is the purpose to test the effectiveness of a nursing intervention designed to reduce preoperative stress? Or is it to learn about the nature of the patients' fears and anxieties? That is, are the patients afraid of the violation of their body boundaries, of loss of control of their body during the anaesthetic, of pain or of the unknown postoperative recovery period?

Answering the first question, the quantitative researcher would make theoretical assumptions using past research about the anxieties of the preoperative patient, and develop an experimental two-group design to measure the effectiveness of the nursing intervention by quantifying differences between the two groups. To answer the second question, the qualitative researcher would describe, in depth, the fears of the preoperative patient in order to understand the experience, and identify a theory of preoperative fears and anxieties.

Following this step the qualitative researcher **may** move into an experimental quantitative research study to test nursing measures which will reduce pre-operative stress.

Occasionally, the choice of qualitative or quantitative measurement will also depend on external resources, such as the expertise of the researcher. Available budget should not influence the researcher's approach but may dictate the size of the project that can be undertaken. Researchers are frequently limited in their choice of research design by the knowledge of their mentor and by their own knowledge, and they are unwilling to try a new approach and new methods.

Unfortunately, funding agencies are also reluctant to fund researchers who do not have a track record using research methods in which they have not previously demonstrated their expertise. A limit on available research funds may also restrict the researcher's choice of methodology.

Qualitative research is comparatively expensive and time-consuming compared to quantitative methods. It is also more difficult to utilize research assistants to conduct unstructured interviews and to assist with data analysis. The researcher must consider the threats to the validity of the research when these constraints dictate the choice of methods and carefully consider the cost of such compromise. However, although the cost of qualitative research is comparatively high, it provides unique insight into the phenomenon being studied   insight that could not be gained any other way.

The maturity of the concept

Maturity of the concept, or how much has already been investigated or is known about the topic, is usually indicated by the amount of information available. If an extensive library search reveals that there is very little previous information about a research topic, then the topic is probably not developed enough to use quantitative methods, and an exploratory, descriptive study using qualitative methods should be conducted. For example if the topic to be investigated is mothers' attitudes towards breast-feeding, there is probably enough literature available on the topic to conduct a quantitative study. But if the research question is, 'What is it like to breast-feed?', where the focus is on the mother's own experience, there is little information available in the literature on this important topic. Thus, a descriptive, qualitative study would be appropriate.

Another occasion in which qualitative methods may be appropriately used is when there is a lot of information available on a particular topic, but a content analysis of the literature reveals that the research is based on assumptions which are not verified or are possibly biased. An example, again from the breast-feeding research, is the assumption that, in order to maintain lactation breasts must be emptied every four hours during the day. This assumption could not be verified in the literature, and a qualitative, exploratory research did not support the assumption (Morse, Harrison and Prowse, 1986).

Therefore qualitative research questions are probably exploratory, seeking to describe a situation or to understand a person or an event (i.e., 'What is ...?' or 'How does ...?' types of questions). If, however, the research question is stated as an hypothesis seeking to demonstrate a relationship between two or more variables, then enough is probably known about the variables to use quantitative methods.

Constraints/confines from the participants or setting

The next factors to consider when selecting methodology arise from characteristics of the participants or the setting. Are the participants literate and, if so, what languages do they speak? Will they be able to read a quantitative questionnaire and, if so, is the questionnaire culturally biased? If, for cultural reasons, quantitative methods are not suitable, then some form of qualitative methods will be necessary. Who are the participants? Are they elderly, disoriented persons or infants? If so, an observational technique, such as ethology, may be more appropriately used than a qualitative interview technique or a quantitative questionnaire.

Researcher characteristics

To a great extent, the method chosen is a product of the researcher. First, the background knowledge and capabilities of the researcher — what the researcher knows is possible and capable of doing — narrows the range of methods considered for the study. If the only qualitative method the researcher knows is grounded theory, for example, then the researcher is likely to design the study that way, or, as Wolcott (1992) a 'dyed-in-the-wool ethnographer' notes, 'recast' the problem ethnographically. While this problem may not be bad, it does restrict the nature of the research and the type of research problem selected. Ideally, the research should be driven by the research question, and appropriate methods should be selected accordingly.

As previously mentioned, research becomes a risky endeavour when driven by the personal agenda of the researcher. When one's own political or personal perspectives override one's ability to view the setting with detachment, the researcher's own agenda may seriously bias and even invalidate the results. Recently, feminists, critical theorists and other interpretative approaches have legitimized the use of such approaches, but for the neophyte researcher, the warning remains. Again, the wise researcher builds a methodological toolbox and develops a critical awareness of self and motives for maximal performance in the research arena.

METHODOLOGICAL THREATS TO VALIDITY

As stated earlier, there is a most appropriate approach to use for each research question. While there are advantages to every method, so there are limitations. Using an inappropriate method to answer a research question may result in loss of generalizability, increased cost and invalidity.

Perhaps the most common problem in the inappropriate use of method is the use of inductive research design and qualitative methods when a considerable amount is known about the topic. Alternatively, it is equally invalid to use deductive research design and quantitative methods when too little is known about the topic. In the first case, researchers develop a conceptual framework and then analyse qualitative data according to the categories in the framework, rather than deriving the categories inductively from the data. Thus, the researcher loses the qualitative strength of validity, by forcing reality to fit the framework. If the researcher knows enough about the topic to be able to create a conceptual framework and identify variables, then the researcher should be using quantitative methods.

The second error is the use of deductive quantitative methods when little is known about the participant. Invalidity occurs when the researchers attempt to create instruments from the literature or their own experience, rather than beginning with a qualitative study to assist with the definition of the concepts. Meaningless, incomplete or erroneous results may be obtained.

In order to conduct valid research, it is imperative that the researcher be aware of personal cultural perspective, bias or agenda. Our example of different cultural interpretations of the same data is Bohannan's (1956/92) account of the interpretation of Shakespeare's *Hamlet* by the Tiv of Africa. Research questions may not be value-free but may even reflect the researcher's cultural values. Morse (1989/92) explores research questions and assumptions that drive infant feeding research and teaching, to illustrate how the theoretical basis of research may be explored.

The first step in becoming a qualitative researcher is to develop an acute sensitivity to the imbedded values and assumptions in society and in present-day theories and research, and an acute awareness of one's own personal values, perspectives and biases. This task is difficult, as many of these values are implicit and not easily recognized until contrasted or challenged by a different norm or set of values. These challenges are most easily identified when the researcher is exposed to another culture, and, for this reason, anthropologists traditionally work cross-culturally.

THINKING QUALITATIVELY

Qualitative questions have particular characteristics. Qualitative inquiry **usually** answers questions pertaining to **what the experience is like**: what it is like to have a particular illness, what it is like to have surgery or to be involved in an accident. Qualitative research is used to describe how groups of people live or how people cope with their daily lives. Qualitative research provides the reader with understanding and enables others to make sense of reality.

While qualitative research may describe phenomena in detail, qualitative research cannot usually be used to answer questions that will prove causality. Neither can it be used to answer questions of 'how much' or 'how many'. Thus, qualitative researchers usually approach a topic or a setting by asking themselves, 'What is going on here?', and systematically exploring the topic or setting as a learner, holding assumptions and knowledge in 'abeyance' until it is confirmed.

Such a value-free approach to research does not imply that such research is atheoretical. Rather, it means that the researcher is not letting theory **drive** the research (Morse, 1992). In a later stage of analysis, when the researcher begins to organize the data and to formulate theory, the researcher compares the findings from the setting with established theory and the results of the research, almost as if drawing a template of others' work over the emerging analysis, to compare the fit. The researcher asks questions constantly about the data: 'Is this interaction supportive?' 'Is this social support?' 'How does this manifestation of social support compare with the definitions in the literature?' 'How is it different?' and 'Why?' The researcher will then expand the sample to include participants who will be able to provide the information necessary to following interesting leads identified in the data.

The interplay between theoretical knowledge and the emerging analysis is interesting. The researcher is always acutely aware of the derivation of an idea — an idea found in the work of others or that is the researcher's own, arising from patterns within the data. The continual comparison of these two levels of information and the multiple decisions that have to be made ('What is **right**, my data or the literature?') force the qualitative researcher to be constantly thinking about his/her project. Thus, qualitative research is an extraordinarily absorbing intellectual exercise; and the good qualitative researcher has a vast knowledge of social science theory, is persistent in fitting the emerging model to both the setting and the literature and never hesitates to redo the analyses.

THE POWER OF QUALITATIVE ENQUIRY

As previously mentioned, qualitative research is inductive. It does not usually have an a priori conceptual framework or hypotheses to be tested. Rather, as the goal is to develop theory, the research must have discovered an interesting **topic**, and be willing and eager to explore it further to learn all about the phenomenon. Recall the outcome of qualitative research is theory. Because the researcher is willing to explore areas that have been relatively neglected by other researchers or to look suspiciously at areas that they believe are perhaps incorrect or in need of modifying, qualitative research has the important role in knowledge development of producing the theory that guides a discipline. Furthermore, because the theory is inductively derived, it is quite likely to be **right**. Thus, qualitative inquiry provides the theory that ideally directs inquiry within a particular discipline.

The developed theory may serve several important functions within a discipline. Firstly, the theory may be applied clinically, either to the setting from which it was developed or to another setting. Thus qualitative research may provide insights that revise or alter clinical practice.

Secondly, qualitative findings provide rich description that enables readers to understand and make sense of clinical reality. It provides a window into the worlds of others, providing empathic understanding of the world. The theory thus enables the readers to make sense of otherwise incomprehensible situations and behaviours. As qualitative theory is data based theory, the theory is more rigorous and valid than theory developed for incomplete data sets or the status quo, and, as such, should be solid enough to withstand external challenge. Thus it directs or redirects the discipline.

Finally, the theory may be used in quantitative research, either as a conceptual framework for quantitative testing, as a basis from which items for psychometric instrument are derived, or triangulated with quantitative findings. Triangulation, in this case, may be either to provide context for the quantitative study or to provide explanation for otherwise unexpected quantitative results.

PRINCIPLES

- The purpose of qualitative research is to construct valid theory that guides knowledge development within a discipline.
- The qualitative perspective is holistic and primarily inductive.
- Research methods must be considered as tools for facilitating inquiry, and so the most appropriate method must be selected to answer the question.
- Excellent researchers are methodologically versatile.
- Qualitative methods are used when little is known about a phenomenon or when present theories need revising.
- The qualitative method chosen should be selected to answer the research question. Other factors to be considered are constraints arising from participants or the setting and the knowledge/attributes of the researcher.
- Qualitative research is a rigorous and time-consuming intellectual endeavour.

REFERENCES

Bohannan, L. (1956/1992) Shakespeare in the bush, in *Qualitative Health Research*, (ed. J.M. Morse), Sage, Newbury Park, CA, pp. 20–30.

Brace, C.L., Gamble, G.R. and Bond, J.T. (eds) (1971) *Race and Intelligence: Anthropological Studies Number 8*, American Anthropological Association, Washington, DC.

Burton, A. (1974) The nature of personality theory, in *Operational Theories of Personality*, (ed. A. Burton), Brunner/Mazel, New York, pp. 1–19.

Chapman, C.R. (1976) Measurement of pain: problems and issues. *Advances in Pain Research and Therapy*, **1**, 345.

Corbin, J. (1986) Coding, writing memos, and diagramming, in *From Practice to Grounded Theory*, (eds W.C. Chenitz and J.M. Swanson), Addison-Wesley, Menlo Park, CA, pp. 91–101.

Duffy, M.E. (1985) Designing nursing research: the qualitative — quantitative debate. *Journal of Advanced Nursing*, **10**, 225–32.

Elliott, M.R. (1983) Maternal infant bonding. *Canadian Nurse*, **79**(8), 28–31.

Engelhardt, H.T. (1974/1992) The disease of masturbation: values and the concept of disease, in *Qualitative Health Research*, (ed. J.M. Morse), Sage, Newbury Park, CA, pp. 5–19.

Feyerabend, P. (1978) *Against Method*, Varo, London.

Geertz, C. (1973) *The Interpretation of Cultures*, Basic Books, New York.

Glaser, B.G. (1978) *Theoretical Sensitivity*, The Sociology Press, Mill Valley, CA.

Glaser, B.G. and Strauss, A.L. (1967) *The Discovery of Grounded Theory: Strategies for Qualitative Research*, Aldine, Chicago.

Goodwin, L.D. and Goodwin, W.L. (1984) Qualitative vs. quantitative research or qualitative and quantitative research? *Nursing Research*, **33**(6), 378–80.

Hinds, P.S., Chaves, D.E. and Cypess, S.M. (1992) Context as a source of meaning and understanding, in *Qualitative Health Research*, (ed. J.M. Morse), Sage, Newbury Park, CA, pp. 31–49.

Klaus, M.H. and Kennel, J.H. (1976) *Parent Infant Bonding: The Impact of Early Separation or Loss on Family Development*, Mosby, St Louis.

Morse, J.M. (1989/1992) 'Euch, those are for your husband!': examination of cultural values and assumptions associated with breastfeeding, in *Qualitative Health Research*, (ed. J.M. Morse), Sage, Newbury Park, CA, pp. 50–60.

Morse, J.M. (1992) If you believe in theories… . *Qualitative Health Research*, **2**(3), 259–61.

Morse, J.M., Harrison, M. and Prowse, M. (1986) Minimal breastfeeding. *Journal of Obstetric Gynecologic and Neonatal Nursing*, **15**(4), 333–8.

Pelto, P.J. and Pelto, G.H. (1978) *Anthropological Research: The Structure of Inquiry*, Cambridge University Press, Cambridge.

Scheper-Hughes, N. (1992) *Death Without Weeping*, University of California Press, Berkeley, CA.

Smith, J.K. (1983) Quantitative versus qualitative research: an attempt to clarify the issue. *Educational Researcher*, **12**(3), 6–13.

Smith, J.K. and Heshusius, L. (1986) Closing down the conversation: the end of the quantitative — qualitative debate among educational inquirers. *Educational Researcher*, **15**, 4–12.

Strauss, A. and Corbin, J. (1990) *Basics of Qualitative Research: Grounded Theory Procedures and Techniques*, Sage, Newbury Park, CA.

Tesch, S. (1981) Disease causality and politics. *Journal of Health Politics, Policy and Law*, **6**(1), 369–89.

Vidich, A.J. and Lyman, S.M. (1994) Qualitative methods: their history in sociology and anthropology, in *Handbook of Qualitative Research*, (eds N.K. Denzin and Y.S. Lincoln), Sage, Newbury Park, CA, pp. 23–59.

Wolcott, H.F. (1992) Posturing in qualitative research, in *The Handbook of Qualitative Research in Education*, (eds M.D. LeCompte, W.L. Millroy and J. Preissle), Academic Press, San Diego, CA, pp. 3–52.

FURTHER READING

Atkinson, P. (1994) Some perils of paradigms. *Qualitative Health Research*, **5**(1).

Denzin, N.K. and Lincoln, Y.S. (eds) (1994) Part II: Major paradigms and perspectives, in *Handbook of Qualitative Research*, Sage, Thousand Oaks, CA, pp. 99–198.

Filstead, W.J. (ed.) (1970) *Qualitative Methodology: Firsthand Involvement with the Social World*, Rand McNally, Chicago.

Gilbert, N. (ed.) (1993) *Researching Social Life*, Sage, London.

Glassner, B. and Moreno, J.D. (eds) (1989) *The Qualitative–Quantitative Distinction in the Social Sciences*, Kluwer, Dordrecht, The Netherlands.

Hammersley, M. (ed) (1993) *Social Research: Philosophy, Politics and Practice*, Sage, London.

Morse, J.M. (ed.) (1992) Part I: The characteristics of qualitative research, in *Qualitative Health Research*, Sage, Newbury Park, CA, pp. 69–90.

Morse, J.M., Bottorff, J.L., Neander, W. *et al.* (1991/1992) Comparative analysis of conceptualizations and theories of caring, in *Qualitative Health Research*, (ed. J.M. Morse), Sage, Newbury Park, CA, pp. 69–90.

Noblit, G.W. and Engel, J.D. (1991/1992) The holistic injunction: an ideal and a moral imperative for qualitative research, in *Qualitative Health Research*, (ed. J.M. Morse), Sage, Newbury Park, CA, pp. 43–63.

Rabinow, P. and Sullivan, W.M. (eds) (1979) *Interpretive Social Science: A Reader*, University of California Press, Berkeley, CA.

Smith, R.B. and Manning, P.K. (eds) (1982) *A Handbook of Social Science Methods*, Ballinger, Cambridge, MA.

An overview of qualitative methods

In the previous chapter, the rationale for a qualitative approach for research was presented. In this chapter, some of the methods that may be used to examine phenomena qualitatively will be introduced, and then factors to consider when selecting a qualitative method will be discussed.

RESEARCH APPROACHES TO STUDYING EVERYDAY EXPERIENCES

Qualitative data have always been used in the social sciences, particularly anthropology, history and political science, but it is only in recent years the qualitative paradigm has developed a role in health care research. Qualitative research is the source of well-grounded theory, illustrated with rich (or thick) description and explanation of processes which occur in an identifiable local context (Miles and Huberman, 1994). When using qualitative approaches, reality is explored from an **emic** perspective, understanding life from the perspective of the participants in the setting under study; and everyday life is examined in an uncontrolled, naturalistic setting. However, life-world structures are viewed in different disciplinary perspectives, which develop in part, from epistemological underpinnings within the main social science disciplines and give rise to distinct methodologies. (These are outlined in Table 2.1). For instance in anthropology, the concept of culture underlies the methods of ethnography and ethnoscience; animal behaviourism and zoology have led to the study of human ethology; ethnomethodology developed from sociology; and phenomenology from applied philosophy.

Phenomenology

The objective of phenomenology is to describe the essence of behaviour, based on meditative thought and with the purpose of promoting human understanding

Table 2.1 Comparison of the major types of qualitative strategies

Type of research questions	Strategy	Paradigm	Method	Other data sources	Major references
Meaning questions — eliciting the essence of experiences	Phenomenology	Philosophy (Phenomenology)	Audiotaped 'conversations'; Written anecdotes of personal experiences	Phenomenological literature; philosophical reflections; poetry; art	Bergum, 1991; Giorgi, 1970; van Manen (1984, 1990)
Descriptive questions — of values, beliefs, practices as a cultural group	Ethnography	Anthropology (Culture)	Unstructured interviews; Participant observation; Fieldnotes	Documents; Records; Photography; Maps; Genealogies; Social network diagrams	Ellen (1984); Fetterman (1989); Grant & Fine (1992); Hammersley & Atkinson (1983); Hughes (1992); Sanjek (1990); Spradley (1979); Werner & Schoepfle (1987a, 1987b)
'Process' questions — experience over time or change, may have stages and phases	Grounded theory	Sociology (Symbolic interactionism)	Interviews (tape recorded)	Participant observation; Memoing; Diary	Glaser & Strauss (1967); Glaser (1978, 1992); Strauss (1987); Strauss & Corbin (1990); Chenitz & Swanson (1986)
Questions regarding verbal interaction and dialogue	Ethnomethodology; Discourse analysis	Semiotics	Dialogue (audio/video recording)	Observation; Fieldnotes	Atkinson (1992); Benson & Hughes (1983); Denzin (1970, 1989); Douglas (1970); Heritage (1984); Leiter (1980); Rogers (1983)
Behavioural questions: Macro	Participant observation	Anthropology	Observation; Fieldnotes	Interviews; Photography	Jorgensen (1989); Spradley (1980)
Micro	Qualitative ethology	Zoology	Observation	Videotape; Note-taking	Eibl-Eibesfeldt (1989); Morse & Bottorff (1990); Scherer & Ekman (1982)

(Source: Morse, J.M. (1994) Designing funded qualitative research, in *Handbook of Qualitative Research*, (eds N.K. Denzin and Y.S. Lincoln), Sage, Thousand Oaks, CA, p. 224. Reprinted with permission of the publisher.)

(Omery, 1983). The phenomenological method is both a philosophy and a method (Cohen, 1987), within which several schools have developed. Cohen and Omery (1994) compare the work of Van Kaam, Colaizzi and Giorgi and explicate the value of each approach for those interested in phenomenology.

The method originated with philosophy, using the work of Husserl, Heidegger, Sartre and Merleau Ponty (van Manen, 1990). The phenomenological tradition seeks to understand the lived experience of individuals and their intention within their 'life-world'. The researcher asks the question, 'What is it like to have a certain experience?' Phenomenology is, therefore, the study of phenomena and the appearance of things, and the discovery of their essence is the ultimate purpose of such research (van Manen, 1990). For example the question might be asked, 'What does it feel like to be a patient receiving chemotherapy?' Data collection may take the form of in-depth conversations in which the researcher and the learner are co-participants.

Omery (1983) notes that it is a requisite of phenomenology that no preconceived notions, expectations or frameworks be present to guide the researchers as they gather and analyse the data. While the life-worlds of individuals being studied are the primary source of data, literature, poetry or art may all be used to gain an understanding of the essence of the phenomena. Unlike grounded theory, where the goal is to develop theory, the goal in the phenomenological method is to provide an accurate description of the phenomena being studied.

Phenomenology accepts experience as it exists in the consciousness of the individual. Phenomenologists maintain that intuition is important in the development of knowledge, although human meaning cannot be inferred from sense impression alone (Bruyn, 1966). Generalization is based on similar meanings rather than on an exact duplication of essence. Phenomenology also does not presuppose the existence of process, although process may be discovered as the research takes place. The goal of phenomenology is to describe accurately the experience of the phenomenon under study and not to generate theories or models, nor to develop general explanation. Some examples from the literature may help to make this point.

Validity rests in the richness of the discussion. Does the description of essence make sense to anyone else? Does it make sense within the context of nursing practice? (Ray, 1994). Phenomenological writing may be descriptive or interpretative, but it is essentially written as text and open to varied interpretation depending on the experience of the reader. Many approaches to qualitative research are classified as 'phenomenology,' if the research focuses on experience. Care must be taken not to take the writer's description of method without question. Kelpin's (1984/92) work on birthing pain reveals pain as a positive experience and provides carers with a new perspective on the meaning of pain in labour. Also Clarke (1990/92) links the child's and the parent's perspectives of a child with asthma in a way that provides insight for the reader.

Ethnography

Historically, ethnography evolved in cultural anthropology and tended to focus on the cultural patterns of village life. Ethnography was incorporated into health care research by nurse-anthropologists, such as Aamodt (1982), Leininger (1969), and Ragucci (1972). This research focused on the effects of culture on health care (Davis, 1986/92), institutions as a cultural setting (Germain, 1979; Golander, 1987/92) or a professional group organized as a cultural system (Cassell, 1987/92).

Recently, Boyle (1994) described a classification system for ethnography under the headings of classical or holistic ethnography, particularistic and focused ethnography, cross-sectional ethnography and ethnohistorical ethnography. She noted that although ethnography may be differentiated by type, most ethnographies share certain common characteristics: they are holistic, contextual, and reflexive. Ethnography is always informed by the concept of culture, and it is a generalized approach to developing concepts and to understanding human behaviours from the insider's point of view. Multiple methods of data gathering are used by the ethnographer, including participant observation, interviews and field-notes, and may be supplemented by other techniques, such as records, chart data, life-histories and so forth.

Ethnography is a means of gaining access to the health beliefs and practices of a culture and allows the observer to view phenomena in the context in which it occurs, thus facilitating our understanding of health and illness behaviour. Such information is critical to the provision of care, for the key to a health programme is through understanding the culture of its recipients. Culture may be used in a broad sense in examining health beliefs of ethnic groups , such as the work by Lipson (1991) on Afghan refugees, or it may also be used to examine the beliefs and practices of delineated communities such as an operating room (Fisher and Peterson, 1993), groups of individuals experiencing a common illness such as a stroke (Häggström, Axelsson and Norberg, 1994), group behavioural norms such as clinical decision making (Stein, 1991) or concepts such as compliance (Roberson, 1992).

An ethnographer asks the question, 'In what ways do members of a community actively construct their world?' Researchers might ask, 'What is it like for a person to live in a nursing home?' The researcher wants to find out whether a person can actively shape his or her life in a nursing home and how they cope in institutions. Another facet of inquiry are the environmental factors that influence coping and adaptation. Differences in perception between the researcher and the subjects can be clarified as they occur and as the researcher gains an understanding of the topic under study from the subject's perspective. Rather than studying people, ethnographers **learn from** people. They set out to grasp the emic or the 'natives' point of view' (Spradley, 1979).

Cassell (1987/92) illustrates this interaction of context and values in her ethnographic study of surgeons. Surgery is based upon critical decision making: the surgeon must therefore be decisive and in control, with emergencies resolved as they occur. The surgeon must remove disease rather than 'out-think and outmanoeuvre it to slow its ravages' (p. 171). Cassell found that surgeons embrace common values related to the occupation which fits them for the profession. Surgeons need a strong ego to survive, but this leads them to a state of paranoia in which they believe everyone and everything is against them, including disease. This suggests that the more certitude surgeons exhibit, the more troubling their inevitable feeling of uncertainty must be — thus the paranoia.

Ideally, ethnographic analysis moves beyond description to reveal or explain aspects of social patterns or observed conduct. Thick description (Geertz, 1973) is an interpretative science that searches for meaning within the cultural norms, culturally patterned behaviour and cultural context, for example in examining Bohannan's (1956/92) article in which she compares a North American interpretation of Shakespeare's *Hamlet* with the interpretation of the Tiv of West Africa. In this article, the differences in the interpretation of the play revealed that the assumptions and rules regarding relationships are cultural-bound and not universal. Thus, the health care researcher is concerned with revealing culturally embedded norms which implicitly guide the actions of individuals in a specific culture, so that the provision of health care may be culturally acceptable.

Grounded theory

Grounded theory was first developed by Glaser and Strauss (1967) to address issues raised within sociology about the understanding of human behaviour based on the quantitative paradigm and statistically average behaviour. The theoretical base for grounded theory is symbolic interactionism. Symbolic interactionism stresses that human behaviour is developed through interaction with others, through continuous processes of negotiation and renegotiation. People construct their own reality from the symbols around them through interaction rather than through a static reaction to symbols. Therefore individuals are active participants in creating meaning in a situation. Grounded theory has as its primary purpose the generation of explanatory theories of human behaviour. Such theory is discovered, developed and then verified through systematic data collection and analysis of data related to an identified phenomenon. Data collection, sampling and analysis all occur simultaneously as the study progresses and sampling and further data collection are based on the emerging theory (Glaser and Strauss, 1967).

In grounded theory, participants are selected based on their knowledge of the topic and on the needs of the developing theory, a process called theoretical sampling (Glaser and Strauss, 1967). Data are generally collected through unstructured interviews, observation and other fieldwork techniques. Analysis techniques include constant comparison, in which all pieces of data are compared with other data. While in ethnography the focus is on cultural beliefs and values, grounded theory is process-oriented and allows for change over time, describing stages and phases inherent in a particular experience.

A grounded theorist may ask the question: 'How do mothers of newly born, hospitalized, preterm infants describe their attachment to their infants over time?' When Brady-Fryer (1994) asked this question, what evolved was a description of how the women coped with 'becoming a mother' in a hospital setting. Lorencz (1991) interviewed in-patients with schizophrenia who were expected to be discharged in the near future. The 'revolving door' patterns of readmission were of concern, and she wanted to understand the hopes and expectations of these patients and their perception of factors leading to admission and readmission. What emerged was a powerful grounded theory explaining the process of 'becoming ordinary'.

Styles of grounded theory As grounded theory has evolved as a research approach, different interpretations have been given to the methods employed. Even the originators of the method appear to have moved in different directions. Stern (1994) presents a useful explanation on the divergence of the method from those originally proposed by Glaser and Strauss. Stern argues that both Glaser and Strauss's studies produce sound work, but that the researcher needs to be clear on what method is being used.

While the literature provides many excellent examples of grounded theory research, one can also find obvious exploratory descriptive studies that deviate from the basic tenets of grounded theory research. What these studies accomplish is a description of what is taking place in the social setting, but they lack conceptualization of the underlying social process at an abstract level and do not 'push' the results towards model development. While these studies are of value, they must also be recognized as limited and not be considered grounded theory.

Qualitative ethology

Ethology is a method of systematically observing, analysing, and describing **behaviours** within the context in which they occur. Ethology was developed and adapted from research on animal behaviour in an attempt to record accurately, describe and derive explanations for the behaviour (Gould, 1982). Ethology has been used in comparative psychology for the study of human behaviour, particularly in the examination of infant behaviour (Blurton-Jones, 1972) and in cross-cultural studies of facial expression (Ekman, Sorenson and Friesen, 1968).

Ethology has been used in the study of human behaviour to identify universal patterns of facial expression (Ekman, 1983) and the behaviour of premature infants (Newman, 1981). Ethology may also be used to explore behaviours in the cognitively impaired, the elderly, the newborn and psychiatric patients (Morse and Bottorff, 1990). Where interviews are inappropriate, it is a useful technique for examining subconscious or transitory phenomena, for example the pain responses of postoperative neonates (Côté, Morse and James, 1991), the touching behaviours of nurses comforting postoperative neonates (Solberg and Morse, 1991), and the nurse's use of touch with oncology patients in pain (Bottorff and Morse, 1994).

In qualitative ethology the actions are recorded on videotape, and patterns of behaviours, antecedents and consequences are subsequently identified. Once the qualitative patterns have been identified, the behavioural scheme (the ethogram) may be quantitatively confirmed by coding time segments and using multivariate statistics such as factor analysis and lag sequential analysis. In this way, complex behavioural patterns and clusters can be elicited from this systematic observation.

Ethnoscience

Ethnoscience (ethnosemantics or ethnolinguistics) was developed in the late 1960s. It evolved as social scientists attempted to increase the rigour of ethnography, which was purported to be 'soft', 'subjective', and 'non-scientific'. Ethnoscience was viewed as a method of developing precise and operationalized descriptions of cultural concepts. As the alternative names ethnosemantics or ethnolinguistics suggest, ethnoscience is derived from linguistics, and researchers employ the structural analysis of phonology and grammar as a basis for data analysis. Basically, it is a method of discovering 'how people can see their world experience from the way they talk about it' (Frake, 1962, p. 74). The goal of the researcher is to describe or comprehend the abstract concept through this analysis, from the perspective of the informants. Thus, cultural systems are determined through the researcher's examination of phenomenological distinctions and those that are significant to the participants themselves.

Levi-Strauss (1963) summarized the process of ethnoscience in the following way:

> The researcher shifts from the analysis of conscious linguistic behaviour to the study of the conscious infrastructure. This process involves examining the relations between terms rather than examining the terms as independent entities. Within the cultural system the purpose of the ethnoscientist is to discover general laws, either by induction or logical deduction.

Ethnoscience interviews will differ from ethnographic interviews or questionnaires on two major dimensions. Firstly, both the questions **and** the answers are 'discovered' or elicited from the participants (Spradley and McCurdy, 1972). Secondly, the meaning of the data is significant from the participant's perspective (that is, it requires emic rather than etic analysis). With questionnaires, statistical analysis gives no interpretation to the meaning of the data or to the organizing principles or relationships of the informant selection of the answer.

The linguistic analysis used in ethnoscience is focused on the **signification**, or the attribution of a concept, and the way in which the attributes are ordered, whereas other linguistics are primarily interested in **connotation**. As an expression also connotes other images or concepts, and these connotations may not be a part of the attributes of the concept, information on the affective or behavioural data may be limited (Goodenough, 1967). The contextual material may, therefore, not be very rich or meaningful when ethnoscience is used alone. In *You Owe Yourself a Drunk*, Spradley (1970) added the contextual dimension by including descriptive letters from his main informant, Bill.

As Evaneshko and Kay (1982) noted, suitable ethnoscience questions are those that answer the 'what' and ultimately, but less directly, the 'why' of cultural behaviour. Ethnoscience questions are most appropriate when identifying the **structure** of a situation is the purpose of the research. For example Morse (1991/92) was interested in the reciprocal nature of care in the patient–nurse relationship, and explored this by examining the types and categories of gifts that patients gave nurses, including retaliative acts given in response to perceived poor care. Note that ethnoscience does not provide affective information; that is, the method does not provide information about how patients feel, only about the categories of gifts.

Ethnomethodology

The purpose of ethnomethodology is to increase the understanding of taken-for-granted or implicit practices in a society. This mode of research had its origins in the sociological research of Garfinkel (1967). Garfinkel's aim was to develop a model of social order built through interpretative work based on ordinary members of society. He believed individuals had the linguistic and interactional competencies to describe the orderly features of everyday reality (Holstein and Gubrium, 1994). The concern is to describe the methods by which people make the social situations in which they are engaged meaningful to themselves and others. In ethnomethodology, the intent is to find how members of society use implicit societal rules to govern their own personal practices, and how they give each other evidence of that social structure (Bowers, 1992).

In an ethnomethodological study, documents and audiovisual material that focus on everyday scenes of life are often the major sources of data. Interviews using stimulated recall are also used. Ethnomethodologists try to show how individuals unknowingly make normative demands on others, implicitly assuming that certain competencies are possessed by others. The general level of the research question is related to unidentified rules which govern conduct; that is 'What taken-for-granted rules do individuals rely on and follow?' An example might be, 'What are the rules which govern patient behaviour that decide that a patient's behaviour is deviant?' In this case, ﹍mpliant individual may determine the rules which are

﹍ted in business and were used to obtain a range of ﹍﹍ on products with the goal of enhancing marketing strategies (Krueger, 1994). One premise related to the use of focus groups is that attitudes and perceptions are not developed in isolation but through interaction with other people. The data obtained in focus groups, while reflecting the views of the individual members, is thus very different from participants' narratives obtained through interviews for grounded theory.

In selecting participants for a focus group, the researcher selects a relatively homogeneous group because the goal in using this technique is to encourage individuals to share their ideas and perceptions. A focus group is typically composed of 7 to 10 participants who are selected because they are known to be knowledgeable about the topic that is focal to the research. Because the purpose in using a focus group is to produce self-disclosure, homogeneity is seen as reducing perceived risk to the informants. For this reason, several focus groups are generally used within a research project to increase the range of beliefs and values that will be represented in the population under study, with the aim to have heterogeneity between the groups.

A global question is used to stimulate discussion. While the researcher may act as facilitator to keep the discussion on topic, it is critical to avoid asking leading questions and taking control of the group interaction. Focus groups allow the researcher to access the attitudes and values of informants while observing the interaction of the participants. The approach is not a substitute for observation in the naturalistic setting since it does not allow for consideration of the context within which the individual's attitudes and values have developed.

Another question that arises is how frequently should the researcher meet with a focus group in order to ensure that all aspects of the phenomenon have been studied? The issue of data saturation within and between groups must also be considered. The advantage of a focus group is that it has been shown to produce believable results at a reasonable price (Krueger, 1994) and it is possible to include a larger number of informants in a study than when one-to-one interviews are used alone. It must be remembered, however, that the purpose of focus groups is to obtain members' opinions about the phenomena of interest. It is not a technique developed to understand the group's culture.

Lankshear (1993) explored the attitudes of teachers to the assessment of student progress. She noted the advantage of talking to a larger group and that members of the group provided support for one another, which she of the data or to the organizing principles or relationships of the informant's selection of the answer.

The linguistic analysis used in ethnoscience is focused on the **signification**, or the attribution of a concept, and the way in which the attributes are ordered, whereas other linguistics are primarily interested in **connotation**. As an expression also connotes other images or concepts, and these connotations may not be a part of the attributes of the concept, information on the affective or behavioural data may be limited (Goodenough, 1967). The contextual material may, therefore, not be very rich or meaningful when ethnoscience is used alone. In *You Owe Yourself a Drunk*, Spradley (1970) added the contextual dimension by including descriptive letters from his main informant, Bill.

As Evaneshko and Kay (1982) noted, suitable ethnoscience questions are those that answer the 'what' and ultimately, but less directly, the 'why' of cultural behaviour. Ethnoscience questions are most appropriate when identifying the **structure** of a situation is the purpose of the research. For example Morse (1991/92) was interested in the reciprocal nature of care in the patient–nurse relationship, and explored this by examining the types and categories of gifts that patients gave nurses, including retaliative acts given in response to perceived poor care. Note that ethnoscience does not provide affective information; that is, the method does not provide information about how patients feel, only about the categories of gifts.

Ethnomethodology

The purpose of ethnomethodology is to increase the understanding of taken-for-granted or implicit practices in a society. This mode of research had its origins in the sociological research of Garfinkel (1967). Garfinkel's aim was to develop a model of social order built through interpretative work based on ordinary members of society. He believed individuals had the linguistic and interactional competencies to describe the orderly features of everyday reality (Holstein and Gubrium, 1994). The concern is to describe the methods by which people make the social situations in which they are engaged meaningful to themselves and others. In ethnomethodology, the intent is to find how members of society use implicit societal rules to govern their own personal practices, and how they give each other evidence of that social structure (Bowers, 1992).

In an ethnomethodological study, documents and audiovisual material that focus on everyday scenes of life are often the major sources of data. Interviews using stimulated recall are also used. Ethnomethodologists try to show how individuals unknowingly make normative demands on others, implicitly assuming that certain competencies are possessed by others. The general level of the research question is related to unidentified rules which govern conduct; that is 'What taken-for-granted rules do individuals rely on and follow?' An example might be, 'What are the rules which govern patient behaviour that enable the nurse to decide that a patient's behaviour is deviant?' In this case, studying the non-compliant individual may determine the rules which are being broken.

Focus groups

Focus groups originated in business and were used to obtain a range of opinions on products with the goal of enhancing marketing strategies (Krueger, 1994). One premise related to the use of focus groups is that attitudes and perceptions are not developed in isolation but through interaction with other people. The data obtained in focus groups, while reflecting the views of the individual members, is thus very different from participants' narratives obtained through interviews for grounded theory.

In selecting participants for a focus group, the researcher selects a relatively homogeneous group because the goal in using this technique is to encourage individuals to share their ideas and perceptions. A focus group is typically composed of 7 to 10 participants who are selected because they are known to be knowledgeable about the topic that is focal to the research. Because the purpose in using a focus group is to produce self-disclosure, homogeneity is seen as reducing perceived risk to the informants. For this reason, several focus groups are generally used within a research project to increase the range of beliefs and values that will be represented in the population under study, with the aim to have heterogeneity between the groups.

A global question is used to stimulate discussion. While the researcher may act as facilitator to keep the discussion on topic, it is critical to avoid asking leading questions and taking control of the group interaction. Focus groups allow the researcher to access the attitudes and values of informants while observing the interaction of the participants. The approach is not a substitute for observation in the naturalistic setting since it does not allow for consideration of the context within which the individual's attitudes and values have developed.

Another question that arises is how frequently should the researcher meet with a focus group in order to ensure that all aspects of the phenomenon have been studied? The issue of data saturation within and between groups must also be considered. The advantage of a focus group is that it has been shown to produce believable results at a reasonable price (Krueger, 1994) and it is possible to include a larger number of informants in a study than when one-to-one interviews are used alone. It must be remembered, however, that the purpose of focus groups is to obtain members' opinions about the phenomena of interest. It is not a technique developed to understand the group's culture.

Lankshear (1993) explored the attitudes of teachers to the assessment of student progress. She noted the advantage of talking to a larger group and that members of the group provided support for one another, which she believed led to a broad expression of feelings and ideas. One problem was that individuals did not always arrive to participate in a scheduled group session, and this resulted in a group of less than optimal size. Transcription was also difficult at times when members interrupted each another or more than one person spoke at the same time. A risk not cited by Lankshear is that one member of a group will often dominate and coerce others into subscribing to a dominant view. This would require intervention by the researcher which could lead to a change of role from facilitator to controller of the discussion.

As with any other method, leadership of a focus group is a skill that must be acquired prior to use in a research study. The technique has promise, but the purpose must be understood and evaluation carried out as it is used in nursing research.

Historical research

The focus of historical research is the interpretation and narration of past events. Most qualitative studies focus on current or ongoing events, so this constitutes the first major difference between qualitative and historical events. In historical research, sources of data are similar to those used in some qualitative work and include documents, records, eyewitness accounts and oral histories. History connects a profession with its heritage and provides a sense of identity, both personally and professionally (Fitzpatrick, 1993), but does not generally focus on the identification of social values. While history describes nursing's relationship to the world, it does so in a general sense rather than establishing the meaning of the world for the individual.

In the **positivistic** or **neo-positivistic** school of historical research, an attempt is made to reduce history to universal laws. Discovery, verification, and categorization of data are used to analyse data, and there is an effort to show cause–effect relationships. Researchers belonging to this school of historical research, while using similar forms of data analysis to qualitative researchers, have very different outcomes in mind. Some survey methods and statistical analyses may also be used to enhance presentation of objective evidence (Fitzpatrick, 1993), and in this respect, too, historical work diverges from pure qualitative methods.

In the **idealist** school, intuition and experience are ingredients for interpretation. From this perspective, historians believe that it is necessary to get inside the event and rethink the thought of the originator in relation to the content of his or her time, place and situation, in order to make adequate historical interpretations (Fitzpatrick, 1993). In comparing this with qualitative research, one must remember that the historian is interpreting past events while the qualitative researcher examines events in the here and now, remembering the effect of history on the context. It is the participants' interpretations of history and its effects, however, that are central to the analysis, rather than the researcher's inference of the effects of earlier events.

Historians use frameworks for analysis in the broad sense. They may examine a Great Person or use a deterministic, sociological, political/economic or psychological framework. In this respect, qualitative researchers will also approach their research with a particular focus. In examining career patterns of nurse-teachers, it is possible that a qualitative researcher will use a sociological framework to support the emerging findings. However, the framework will not be determined prior to the analysis.

Finally, one can argue that all historical research is chronological and presents events over a specified period of time; it is the interpretation of the data within context that makes it unique. Thus, while qualitative research and historical research have some common areas of data sources and analysis, their goals and purposes differ, and they are two distinct traditions which require different training and mentoring.

SELECTING A METHOD

Given, then, that the problem is best studied by using a qualitative approach, how does a researcher select the 'best' or the most appropriate method? Again, it depends upon what one wishes to know, what the expected outcomes of the research will be, the constraints of the setting, the subjects and, to a lesser extent, on the resources available to the researcher.

The difference between the major qualitative methods, the different kinds of questions that they answer, the different methodological requirements and the different types of results are shown in Table 2.2. This table was constructed for a hypothetical project called, 'Arrivals and departures: patterns of human attachment', in which students are asked to image how a research study would be conducted at an international airport (Morse, 1994).

If the purpose of the research is to describe a setting or a community, then ethnography (that is interviews combined with participant observation) would be appropriate. But if the purpose is to describe the types of health care professionals in the community, then the question becomes more suited to an ethnoscience approach. Phenomenology would answer experiential questions such as 'What does it feel like to be a patient?' Finally, participant observation alone may be used to examine the behaviours of the people in the community as they 'become patients' in the waiting room of the hospital. For each question, there is a best or most appropriate method, and selecting the method is the most important decision in the research process.

PRINCIPLES

- The primary purpose of qualitative research is to develop rich descriptions and valid theory.

Table 2.2 A comparison of strategies in the conduct of a hypothetical project, 'Arrivals and departures: patterns of human attachment'

Strategy	Research question/focus	Participants/ informants*	Sample size†	Data collection methods	Type of results
Phenomenology	What is the meaning of arriving home?	Travellers arriving home Phenomenological literature Art, poetry and other descriptions	Approx. six participants	In-depth conversations	In-depth reflective description of the experience, 'What does it feel like to come home?'
Ethnography	What is the arrival gate like when an international plane arrives?	Travellers, families; others who observe the setting, such as porters, rental car personnel, cleaning staff, security guards and so forth	Approx. 30–50 interviews	Interviews Participant observation Other records, such as airport statistics	Description of the day-to-day events at the arrival gate of the airport
Grounded theory	Coming home: Reuniting the family	Travellers, family members	Approx. 30–50	In-depth interviews Observations	Description of the social psychological process in the experience of returning home
Ethnoscience	What are types of travellers	Those who observe the setting daily — porters, rental car personnel, cleaning staff, security guards and so forth	Approx. 30–50	Interviews to elicit similarities and differences of travellers Card sorts	Taxonomy and description of types and characteristics of travellers
Qualitative Ethology	What are the greeting behaviours of travellers and their families?	Travellers and their families	Units — numbers of greetings — 100–200	Photography Video Coded	Description of the patterns of greeting behaviours

(Source: Morse, J.M., (1994) Designing funded qualitative research, in *Handbook of Qualitative Research*, (eds N.K. Denzin and Y.S. Lincoln), Sage, Thousand Oaks, CA, p. 255. Reprinted with permission of the publisher.)
* Examples only
† Number depends on saturation

- Major methods include phenomenology, grounded theory, ethnography, qualitative ethology, ethnoscience and focus groups.
- Each of the qualitative methods answers different questions; the methods are distinct and the results provide a different perspective of the phenomenon.

REFERENCES

Aamodt, A.M. (1982) Examining ethnography for nurse researchers. *Western Journal of Nursing Research*, **4**(2), 209–21.

Atkinson, P. (1992) The ethnography of a medical setting: reading, writing and rhetoric. *Qualitative Health Research*, **2**, 451–74.

Benson, D. and Hughes, J.A. (1983) *The Perspective of Ethnomethodology*, Longman, London.

Bergum, V. (1991) Being a phenomenological researcher, in *Qualitative Nursing Research: A Contemporary Dialogue*, (ed. J.M. Morse), Sage, Newbury Park, CA, pp. 55–71.

Blurton-Jones, N.G. (1972) Characteristics of ethological studies of human behaviour, in *Ethological Studies of Childhood Behaviour*, (ed. N. Blurton-Jones), Cambridge University Press, Cambridge, England, pp. 3–33.

Bohannan, L. (1956/1992) Shakespeare in the bush, in *Qualitative Health Research*, (ed. J.M. Morse), Sage, Newbury Park, CA, pp. 20–30.

Bottorff, J.L. and Morse, J.M. (1994) Identifying types of attending: patterns of nurses' work. *Image: Journal of Nursing Scholarship*, **26**(1), 53–60.

Bowers, L. (1992) Ethnomethodology I: an approach to nursing research. *International Journal of Nursing Studies*, **29**(1), 59–68.

Boyle, J. (1994) Style of ethnograph, in *Critical Issues in Qualitative Research Methods*, (ed. J.M. Morse), Sage, Thousand Oaks, CA, pp. 159–85.

Brady-Fryer, B. (1994) Becoming the mother of a preterm baby, in *Uncertain Motherhood: Negotiating Risk in the Childbearing Years*, (eds P.A. Field and P.B. Marck), Sage, Thousand Oaks, CA, pp. 195–222.

Bruyn, S.R. (1966) *The Human Perspective in Sociology*, Prentice Hall, Englewood Cliffs, NJ.

Cassell, J. (1987/92) On control, certitude and the 'paranoia' of surgeons, in *Qualitative Health Research*, (ed. J.M. Morse), Sage, Newbury Park, CA, pp. 170–91.

Chenitz, W.C. and Swanson, J.M. (1986) *From Practice to Grounded Theory*, Addison-Wesley, Menlo Park, CA.

Clarke, M. (1990/92) Memories of breathing: a phenomenological dialogue: Asthma as a way of becoming, in *Qualitative Health Research*, (ed. J.M. Morse), Sage, Newbury Park, CA, pp. 123–40.

Cohen, M.Z. (1987) A historical overview of the phenomenological movement. *Image: Journal of Nursing Scholarship*, **19**, 31–4.

Cohen, M.Z. and Omery, A. (1994) Schools of phenomenology: implications for research, in *Critical Issues in Qualitative Research Methods*, (ed. J.M. Morse), Sage, Thousand Oaks, CA, pp. 136–57.

Côté, J.J., Morse, J.M. and James, S.G. (1991) The pain response of the postoperative newborn. *Journal of Advanced Nursing*, **16**(4), 378–87.

Davis, D.L. (1986/92) The meaning of menopause in a Newfoundland fishing village, in *Qualitative Health Research*, (ed. J.M. Morse), Sage, Newbury Park, CA, pp. 145–69.

Denzin, N.K. (1970). Symbolic interactionism and ethnomethodology, in *Understanding Everyday Life*, (ed. J. Douglas), Aldine, NY, pp. 261–86.

Denzin, N.K. (1989) *Interpretive Interactionism*, Newbury Park, Sage, CA.

Douglas, J. (1970) *Understanding Everyday Life*, Aldine, Chicago, IL.

Eibl-Eibesfeldt, I. (1989) *Human Ethology*, Aldine de Gruyter, New York.

Ekman, P. (ed.) (1983) *Emotion in the Human Face*, 2nd edn, Cambridge University Press, Cambridge.

Ekman, P., Sorenson, E.R. and Friesen, W.V. (1968) Pan-cultural elements in facial displays of emotions. *Science*, **164**, 86–8.

Ellen, R.F. (ed.) (1984) *Ethnographic research*, Academic Press, London.

Evaneshko, V. and Kay, M.A. (1982) The ethnoscience research technique. *Western Journal of Nursing Research*, **4**(1), 49–64.

Fetterman, D.M. (1989) *Ethnography: Step by Step*, Sage, Melno Park, CA.

Fisher, B.J. and Peterson, C. (1993) She won't be dancing much anyway: A study of surgeons, surgical nurses and elderly patients. *Qualitative Health Research*, 3, 165–83.

Fitzpatrick, M.L. (1993) Historical research, in *Nursing Research: A Qualitative Perspective*, 2nd edn, (eds P.L. Munhall and C.O. Boyd), National League for Nursing, New York, pp. 359–90.

Frake, C.O. (1962) The ethnographic study of cognitive systems, in *Anthropology and Human Behavior*, (eds T. Gladwin and W.C. Sturveant), Anthropological Society of Washington, Washington, DC, pp. 72–85.

Garfinkel, H. (1967) *Studies in Ethnomethodology*, Prentice-Hall, Englewood Cliffs, NJ.

Geertz, C. (1973) *The Interpretation of Cultures*, Basic Books, New York.

Germain, C. (1979) *The Cancer Unit: An Ethnography*, Nursing Resources, Wakefield, MA.

Giorgi, A. (1970) *Psychology As A Human Science: A Phenomenologically Based Approach*, Harper and Row, New York.

Glaser, B.G. (1978) *Theoretical Sensitivity*, The Sociology Press, Mill Valley, CA.

Glaser, B.G. (1992) *Basics of Grounded Theory Analysis*, The Sociology Press, Mill Valley, CA.

Glaser, B.G. and Strauss, A.L. (1967) *The Discovery of Grounded Theory: Strategies for Qualitative Research*, Aldine, New York.

Golander, H. (1987/92) Under the guide of passivity, in *Qualitative Health Research*, (ed. J. Morse), Sage, Newbury Park, CA, pp. 192–201.

Goodenough, W.H. (1967) Componential analysis. *Science*, **156**, 1203–09.

Gould, J.L. (1982) *Ethology*, W.W. Norton and Company, London.

Grant, L. and Fine, G.A. (1992) Sociology unleashed: creative directions in classical ethnography, in *The Handbook of Qualitative Methodology*, (eds M.D. LeCompte, W.L. Millroy and J. Preissle), Academic Press, San Diego, CA, pp. 405–46.

Häggström, M.T., Axelsson, K. And Norberg, A. (1994) The experience of living with stroke sequelae illuminated by means of stories and metaphors. *Qualitative Health Research*, **4**(3), 321–37.

Hammersley, M. and Atkinson, P. (1983) *Ethnography: Principles in Practice*, Tavistock, London.

Heritage, J. (1984) *Garfinkel and Ethnomethodology*, Polity Press, Cambridge.

Holstein, J.A. and Gubrium, J.F. (1994) Phenomenology, ethnomethodology and interpretive practice, in *Handbook of Qualitative Research*, (eds N.K. Denzin and Y.S. Lincoln), Sage, Thousand Oaks, CA, pp. 262–72.

Hughes, C.C. (1992) 'Ethnography': what's in a work — process? product? promise? *Qualitative Health Research*, **2**, 451–74.

Jorgensen, D.L. (1989) *Participant Observation: A Methodology for Human Studies*, Sage, Newbury Park, CA.

Kelpin, V. (1984/92) Birthing pain, in *Qualitative Health Research*, (ed. J.M. Morse), Sage, Newbury Park, CA, pp. 93–103.

Krueger, R.A. (1994) *Focus Groups*, 2nd edn, Sage, Thousand Oaks, CA.

Lankshear, A.J. (1993) The use of focus groups in a study of attitudes to student nurses assessment. *Journal of Advanced Nursing*, **18**, 1986–9.

Leininger, M. (1969) Ethnoscience: a promising research approach to improve nursing practice. *Image: The Journal of Nursing Scholarship*, **3**(1), 2–8.

Leiter, K. (1980) *A Primer on Ethnomethodology*, Oxford University Press, New York.

Levi-Strauss, C. (1963) *Structural Anthropology*, Basic Books, New York.

Lipson, J.G. (1991) The use of self in ethnographic research, in *Qualitative Nursing Research*, (ed. J.M. Morse), Sage, Newbury Park, CA, pp. 73–89.

Lorencz, B. (1991) Becoming ordinary: leaving the psychiatric hospital, in *The Illness Experience: Dimensions of Suffering*, (eds J.M. Morse and J. Johnson), Sage, Newbury Park, CA, pp. 140–200.

Miles, M.B. and Huberman, A.M. (1994) *Qualitative Data Analysis*, Sage, Thousand Oaks, CA.

Morse, J.M. (1991/92) The structure and function of gift-giving in the patient — nurse relationship, in *Qualitative Health Research*, (ed. J.M. Morse), Sage, Newbury Park, CA, pp. 236–56.

Morse, J.M. (1994) Designing funded qualitative research, in *Handbook of Qualitative Research*, (eds N.K. Denzin and Y.S. Lincoln), Sage, Thousand Oaks, CA, pp. 220–35.

Morse, J.M. and Bottorff, J. (1990) The use of ethology in clinical nursing. *Advances in Nursing Science*, **12**(3), 53–64.

Newman, L.F. (1981, April 13) *Anthropology and ethology in the special care nursery: communicative functions in low birthweight infants*, paper presented to the Society for Applied Anthropology, Edinburgh, Scotland.

Omery, A. (1983) Phenomenology: a method for nursing research. *Advances in Nursing Science*, **5**, 49–63.

Ragucci, A. (1972) The ethnographic approach to nursing research. *Nursing Research*, **21**, 485–90.

Ray, M.A. (1994) The richness of phenomenology: philosophic, theoretic and methodologic concerns, in *Critical Issues in Qualitative Research*, (ed. J.M. Morse), Sage, Thousand Oaks, CA, pp. 117–33.

Roberson, M.H.B. (1992) The meaning of compliance: patient perspectives. *Qualitative Health Research*, **2**(1), 7–26.

Rogers, M. F. (1983) *Sociology, Ethnomethodology, and Experience*, Cambridge University Press, Cambridge.

Sanjek, R. (1990) *Fieldnotes: The Makings of Anthropology*, Cornell University Press, Ithica, NY.

Scherer, K.R. and Ekman, P. (1982) *Handbook of Methods in Nonverbal Behavior Research*, Cambridge University Press, Cambridge, MA.

Solberg, S. and Morse, J.M. (1991) The comforting behaviors of caregivers toward distressed postoperative neonates. *Issues in Comprehensive Pediatric Nursing*, **14**, 77–92.

Spradley, J.P. (1970) *You Owe Yourself a Drunk: An Ethnography of Urban Nomads*, Little, Brown and Company, Boston.

Spradley, J.P. (1979) *The Ethnographic Interview*, Holt, Rinehart and Winston, New York.

Spradley, J.P. (1980) *Participant Observation*, Holt, Rinehart and Winston, New York.

Spradley, J.P. and McCurdy, D. (1972) *The Cultural Experience: Ethnography in Complex Society*, Science Research Associates, Chicago.

Stein, H.F. (1991) The role of some nonbiomedical parameters in clinical decision making: an ethnographic approach. *Qualitative Health Research*, **1**, 6–26.

Stern, P.N. (1994) Eroding grounded theory, in *Critical Issues in Qualitative Research Methods*, (ed. J.M. Morse), Sage, Thousand Oaks, CA, pp. 212–23.

Strauss, B.G. (1987) *Qualitative Data Analysis for Social Scientists*, Cambridge University Press, Cambridge.

Strauss, A. and Corbin, J. (1990) *Basics of Qualitative Research*, Sage: Newbury Park, CA.

van Manen, M. (1984) Practicing phenomenological writing. *Phenomenology and Pedagogy*, **2**, 36–69.

van Manen, M. (1990) *Researching Lived Experience*, The Althouse Press, London, Ont.

Werner, O. and Schoepfle, G.M. (1987a) *Systematic Fieldwork: Foundations of Ethnography and Interviewing (Vol. 1)*, Sage, Newbury Park, CA.

Werner, O. and Schoepfle, G.M. (1987b) *Systematic Fieldwork: Ethnographic Analysis and Data Management (Vol. 2)*, Sage, Newbury Park, CA.

FURTHER READING

Aessler, D.C. and Tomlinson, P.S. (1988) Nursing research and the discipline of ethological science. *Western Journal of Nursing Research*, **10**, 743–56.

Allen, M. and Jensen, L. (1990) Hermeneutical inquiry: meaning and scope. *Western Journal of Nursing Research*, **12**, 241–53.

Becker, P.H. (1993) Common pitfalls in published grounded theory research. *Qualitative Health Research*, **3**, 254–60.

Cressler, D.L. and Tomlinson, P.S. (1988) Nursing research and the discipline of ethological science. *Western Journal of Nursing Research*, **10**(6), 743–56.

Davis, A.J. (1978) The phenomenological approach in nursing research, in *The Nursing Profession: Views Through the Mist*, (ed. N.L. Chaska), McGraw-Hill, New York, pp. 186–96.

Gilgun, J.F., Daly, K. and Handel, G. (eds) (1992) *Qualitative Methods in Family Research*, Sage, Newbury Park, CA.

Goodwin, L.D. and Goodwin, W.L. (1984) Qualitative vs. quantitative research or qualitative and quantitative research. *Nursing Research*, **33**, 378–80.

Gubrium, J.F. and Sankar, A. (eds) (1994) *Qualitative Methods in Aging Research*, Sage, Thousand Oaks, CA.

Hughes, C.C. (1992) 'Ethnography' What's in a word — process? product? promise? *Qualitative Health Research*, **2**, 439–50.

Mitchell, E.S. (1986) Multiple triangulation: a methodology for nursing science. *Advances in Nursing Science*, **8**, 18–26.

Morgan, D.L. (1988) *Focus Groups as Qualitative Research*, Sage, Newbury Park, CA.

Munhall, P.L. (1989) Philosophical ponderings on qualitative research methods in nursing. *Nursing Science Quarterly*, **2**, 20–8.

Robertson, H.B. and Boyle, J.S. (1984) Ethnography: contributions to nursing research. *Journal of Advanced Nursing*, **9**, 43–50.

Silverman, D. (1985) *Qualitative Methodology and Sociology*, Gower, Hants, England.

Spradley, J.P. (1979) *The Ethnographic Interview*, Holt, Rinehart and Winston, Orlando.

Stern, P.N. (1994) Eroding grounded theory, in *Critical Issues in Qualitative Research*, (ed. J.M. Morse), Sage, Thousand Oaks, CA, pp. 212–23.

Swanson-Kaufman, K. (1986) A combined methodology for nursing research. *Advances in Nursing Science*, **8**, 58–69.

Taylor, B. (1993) Phenomenology: one way to understanding nursing practice. *International Journal of Nursing Studies*, **30**, 171–9.

van Maanen, J., Dabbs, J.M., Jr and Faulkner, R.R. (1982) *Varieties of Qualitative Research*, Sage, Beverly Hills, CA.

Werner, O. (1994) Short take 12: ethnoscience 1994. *Cultural Anthropology Methods*, February 1994, **6**, pp. 5–8.

Principles of conceptualizing a qualitative project | 3

When preparing a qualitative research proposal, researchers often find themselves in a paradoxical situation. Researchers have deliberately selected a qualitative method because little is known about the area — yet how can they write about, for instance how they are going to analyse data when the nature of these data are not known? How can a qualitative researcher convince a funding agency that a study is worthwhile when so much is unknown? Whereas **quantitative** research proposals are generally highly structured and serve to guide the research process, it is not possible to develop a rigid protocol for a **qualitative** research proposal while still remaining true to the principles of qualitative inquiry. While the quantitative proposal may serve as an indicator that the student is ready to collect data, has identified a theoretical framework and has a sound protocol for data analysis, the qualitative proposal serves only to convince the committee that the topic is worth studying. Despite the fact that the qualitative researcher may not know very much about the research topic or what will be found out, she or he must entice the committee in order to be allowed to proceed. This lack of development may be a handicap if the qualitative proposal is to be submitted to a funding agency, and the onus is on the researcher to convince the granting agency that funding the research is 'a good risk.'

Clearly, developing a rigid plan for a qualitative project, including detailed plans for data collection and analysis, becomes impossible when writing qualitative proposals. The problem is that qualitative researchers often **select** a topic because little is known about it. Therefore, the literature is too scant to develop a theoretical framework or testable hypotheses. Remember, the purpose of conducting the study is to find out about the phenomenon. Furthermore, because there are no tests that can be used to estimate sample size (and the number of participants depends on the quality of the interviews, the broadness of the topic and complexity of the setting), qualitative researchers cannot predetermine the sample size and consequently cannot state the number of interviews and budget the costs for transcription. Neither can the investigator often know what questions will be asked of participants. Investigators may be unsure about what the setting will be like, how quickly the research may gain trust and whether they will be able to collect data effectively and efficiently. Finally, it is hard to justify the significance of the research findings, and the researcher cannot, with confidence, make assurances to the granting agency that the results will be important — only that the results will be interesting. In this chapter, the process of preparing to do qualitative research and the components of a qualitative research proposal will be described.

THE QUALITATIVE PROPOSAL

Identifying the topic

The first step in preparing to do research is to decide on the research topic and to define the research problem. As we have mentioned, qualitative research is used for particular types of problems, the most common use being when little is known about the topic. Other characteristics such as the purpose of the research or the nature of the research question are also important. For example it is appropriate to use qualitative methods when you are needing to ask: 'What is going on here?', 'How do these people feel when ...?', and 'What is important when ...?' On the other hand, it is not appropriate to use qualitative methods if all the variables are identified. 'How many people feel this way?' or 'What is the relationship between ... and ...?' are quantitative questions, demanding how much and how many. Quantitative methods are more appropriately used to measure the distribution of a phenomenon such as attitudes or to confirm relationships between variables.

How does a new researcher decide on a topic? One approach is to do some self-reflection to identify what are the topics that he or she considers most interesting. The researcher should ask: 'What articles catch my eye when I am working in the library?'; 'What topics do I constantly think about and often discuss in general conversation?' Carefully consider extraordinary experiences that have occurred in clinical practice. Perhaps you had contact with a particularly interesting patient who forced you to re-examine conventional ideas about appropriate care. Or recall a clinical observation that was not documented in the literature. Or perhaps there have been recommendations in the patient care literature that are not in agreement with practice. Researchers often find topics within these areas that are particularly intriguing or interesting. Researchers may find research questions in conversation with others or by reading lay accounts of the illness experience or biographies. Finding a topic takes some self-examination, and the discussion of one's ideas with colleagues and experienced qualitative researchers is essential. The researcher must find the topic chosen to be fascinating, for to work for six months or a year on a topic that is boring converts what should be an exciting activity into drudgery.

At this stage the topic selected is very general. There may or may not be a definite research question identified — it does not matter at this point, for, at this preliminary stage, the next step is to find out what is already known about the topic.

Exploring the literature

There are some differences of opinion amongst qualitative researchers about the extent to which the literature should be used to guide qualitative research. There are three main viewpoints on this issue. The first view, recommended for grounded theory by Glaser (1978, p. 31), is that the researcher does not consult the literature prior to conducting fieldwork. The main argument for this position is that the literature may mislead or distract the researcher's perception and ability to make accurate and value-free decisions in the setting. Researchers subscribing to this position, therefore, attempt to enter the setting uninformed, thus minimizing the risk of working deductively. The obvious disadvantage of this approach is that an extraordinary amount of time is spent 'reinventing the wheel' or rediscovering facts that are already published research.

The second point of view is that one should locate, read, and utilize all information available on the research topic. Frequently this is not an extensive body of literature, therefore this may not be an immense task. The important point is that all the major literature is incorporated into the **literature review** portion of the proposal. When beginning data collection, the researcher holds this knowledge 'in abeyance' or brackets others' theories to minimize the threat to validity extending from unconsciously working deductively. Nevertheless, the researcher risks losing control when using this method, for example van Gennep (1967/92) provides an interesting illustration in which a graduate became immersed in the library seeking obscure references. Previous research may be based on false or biased assumptions distorting the present, or the setting may have changed over time so that the reality has altered since the previous research was conducted.

The third method, which we recommend, is to examine previous research critically and to use this work selectively. This involves obtaining all relevant literature and conducting an extensive content analysis, examining all the literature for explicit and implicit assumptions, for biases in measurement and unsubstantiated conclusions. Finally, as all settings are not the same and changes may occur over time, this literature may be used to **guide** the researcher into assisting with deriving explanations from previous research results or prevailing theories. By using this method the researchers are open and informed, but this knowledge does not restrict the researcher's ability to analyse the setting by trying to fit reality into a conscious or unconscious 'framework' developed from previously published analyses.

Selecting the setting

Before writing the research proposal, it is a good idea to try to locate a setting in which to conduct your research. The setting chosen should give the researcher the opportunity to observe the research topic, therefore select a setting that both maximizes the intensity of the phenomenon that you wish to study and the frequency that the phenomenon occurs. For instance do not study pain in a setting in which pain is well controlled with analgesics. Go to a setting in which pain is maximized, such as a cardiac catheterization, a trauma room or a labour and delivery suite. Because the proposal should be tailored to a particular setting, visit the selected site on a preliminary basis and informally get the cooperation and permission of the staff to host the study. Formal permission should be sought in the approval process when the proposal is completed.

Writing the proposal

A qualitative proposal is an argument, a persuasive argument that convinces the reader that a particular topic is worth exploring. The trick is to draw the reader into believing that the topic you want to study is fascinating, significant and will answer many critical questions. There must be an urgency about the proposal, so that by the time the reader has read the literature review, the reader will feel it is imperative that the study be conducted.

The qualitative proposal must achieve two objectives: convince the reader that the study is significant, and convince the reader that the investigator knows how to do and is capable of doing the research. Firstly, the qualitative proposal is thus argued as a political statement. This does not mean that some of the literature is ignored — all pertinent literature should be addressed — rather, the structure of the argument makes a case for the significance of the study. The argument moves logically from the general to the specific, asks questions of the reader, points out holes in current thinking and often attacks basic values and assumptions or the theoretical underpinnings of the field. The language used does not have to be entirely the value-free language normally used in science, and the proposal must be interesting and lively.

Secondly, convince the reader that you, as an investigator, know how to do qualitative research. If you have conducted previous studies, make sure that your experience as a researcher is noted, either in the literature review as 'previous studies' or background work, under the section describing the investigator, or weave this information into the methods section ('In my experience ...'). Presume the reader will know very little of qualitative methods, so few unidentified terms are used and the methods section is clear and detailed. When writing about data analysis, insert a paragraph of text and demonstrate how it will be coded. If you do not have any data, then select a paragraph of text from a biography or make something up — simply noting the source and that it is confabulated data. But do not waste this space. This is an opportunity for you to insert a 'human touch' in your proposal, so be certain to select something that will touch the heartstrings of even the most stony reviewer.

An example of a proposal is presented in Appendix A. Note how the proposal begins by asking a question ('What is comfort?'), so that the reader is immediately and actively drawn into the inquiry. The purpose of that project was to try to discern what comfort was, so in the proposal the researcher tried to make the reader realize that although comfort was an everyday concept, there was much that was not understood about it, much to be learned and the concept could be very important for nursing. The reviewers' report is presented in Appendix B , and the way a qualitative proposal is reviewed is apparent in this report. Most of the 'weight' of the review is on the topic, rather than on the methods *per se*. These reviewers were concerned that: (1) the study was important or worth doing; (2) that the investigator knew what she/he was talking about — a criteria that denotes the folly of not doing library work at this stage; and (3) that the investigator would know how to conduct the study methodologically.

Every proposal is tailored to the requirements of the reader. If the 'reader' is a funding agency, then obtain a copy of their guidelines and, if possible, a proposal that has previously been funded by that agency. Follow their guidelines meticulously; to exceed that page limit or to omit required information may result in the proposal not being reviewed. If the proposal is to meet departmental and university requirements for a thesis or dissertation, again produce what the committee wants and expects. In this case, these proposals become Chapter 1 (Introduction), Chapter 2 (Literature review), and Chapter 3 (Methods) of the finished document. However, while this organizational plan is appropriate for quantitative research, it is not without risks for the qualitative project because, when the qualitative study is completed, the Literature review (Chapter 2) and the Introduction (Chapter 1) may not be a good fit and may have to be rewritten. When the study is completed, if these two chapters remain suitable to be used for the actual thesis/dissertation, then all is well. But do not keep these chapters intact simply because they have been written. It is more likely that these chapters will need to be rewritten, and that the focus of the study will have changed dramatically when the researcher really learns about the topic following data collection and analysis. Do not let the proposal 'drive' the study, for that, in itself, will introduce a threat to validity. In the next section, each of the components of a proposal will be described, and the ways to make the proposal as strong as possible will be identified.

Cover page

All formal documents have a cover page that introduces the document. Sometimes a cover page is provided by the funding agency and is a part of several pages of forms in which identifying information is requested. Otherwise, the investigator should create a cover page, listing:

- title of the proposal;
- name and affiliation of the principal investigator and co-investigators;
- signature line for the principal investigator and university signatories, if relevant;
- contact information — address, phone and fax numbers, and e-mail address;
- name of the agency (and possibly the department or committee) to which the proposal is to be submitted.

The proposal may be regarded as a promissory note between the researcher and the funding agency. That is there is an 'agreement' that, if the research is funded by the agency, the researcher will conduct the project more or less as outlined in the proposal. This may place qualitative researchers in an awkward position, because the qualitative proposal must be written to give the investigator some room to investigate the topic. However, after the grant is awarded, if major changes in the research design are required, the granting agency must be informed and the changes negotiated and approved.

The abstract

The abstract is a concise summary of the proposal, yet it must be comprehensive enough to inform the review committee and to introduce the project. It usually begins with a general statement of the problem and then summarizes the importance of the problem and the method to be used. The plan for data analysis methods must be briefly described. The length of the abstract will be dictated by the funding agency's guidelines, but usually does not exceed 200 words. Remember: the abstract is the first part of the proposal that the reader will read, is the part of the proposal that is submitted to the agency's Board of Directors for approval and is often published by the granting agency to show the type of work they are funding — therefore, spend some time on the abstract and make it a strong statement.

Because of the above pressures, the abstract is the most frequent cause of writer's block. But, as it is not possible to write the abstract until you have written what you are going to do, leave the writing of the abstract until last. At that time the abstract will be much easier to write.

The body of the proposal

The proposal should begin with an introduction or a short passage explaining the problem and justifying the need for the study. This section should grab the attention, and convince the reader that this is a significant and unique topic to study. This section may end with a formal summary under the heading,

Statement of the problem. Under a subheading, **Delimitations of the study**, the anticipated limitations of the projected research project should be listed. If necessary, all less familiar terms, or terms that will be used in a particular way, may be listed in alphabetical order and defined in a section titled, Definition of terms. As the purpose of this section is to orientate the reader, do not list terms that are obvious, basic or common. Because the qualitative researcher does not operationalize variables, this section is not required very often, and definitions can often be woven into the text.

Literature review

As stated previously, this section must be written to convince the reviewer that the study is worthwhile. Previous research is critiqued, and the researcher demonstrates how the present project will clarify or compensate for shortcomings in previous research and how the study will add to present knowledge. The argument must be constructed moving from the general to the specific and should justify the selection of the topic and the research setting or selection of participants, ending with the research question.

The literature review should also contain a short section in which the **Implications** of the study are discussed. Why will the study be important? This question enables the reviewer to evaluate the need for the research and the pragmatic implications of the study. This is particularly important when the contribution to knowledge is perhaps obscure. For example Morse examined gift-giving in hospitals. While the importance of this topic may have appeared obscure to a review committee, **if** the argument can be presented that gift-giving was an indicator of reciprocity for care, quality of care and patient satisfactions, and was, perhaps, a phenomenon that decreased patient passivity and dependency and nurse burn out, then the importance of the research becomes more obvious. In the 'Comfort' proposal (Appendix A), the significance was argued in terms of the theoretical shift from the nurse to the patient, so that the outcomes of comforting interventions could then possibly be measured. Note that this type of argument is different from a conceptual framework, in that it provides a theoretical context for the study *per se* but does not drive the study or provide an outline for analysis, as does a conceptual framework. Establishing a theoretical context for the study does not identify the variables nor dictate the relationship between variables, as would be the case with a theoretical framework for a quantitative design.

Methods

The **Methods** section starts with a short description of the setting in which the research will be conducted. Describe the setting in detail and explain why this setting was selected. If the planned study is an ethnography or other design in which the structure of the setting is important, include a floor plan. Present evidence that the agency or staff knows about the study and has approved of the study being conducted at the site by including letters of agreement from administration and letters of support from key staff members.

Describing the sample — for example who will be interviewed and how many interviews there will be — is a problem for the qualitative researcher because the number and type of participants cannot be predicted at the beginning of the study. Yet such information is crucial for calculating the budget and so forth. Perhaps the only way to manage this problem is to generously estimate the number of participants and to justify why the exact number cannot be calculated in the proposal. The fact that qualitative researchers cannot know in advance exact details, such as sample size, may not be apparent to reviewers, so cite several sources that support this argument. Such straightforwardness is a sign of a good researcher and, as long as a clear rationale is presented, such detail will actually work for the researcher rather than against. Review committees are now becoming suspicious of qualitative proposals that are written with dogmatic preciseness.

Procedures used in the research must be explained in detail. Agar (1980) notes that it is inadequate to simply write that data will be collected using 'participant observation, fieldnotes, and diary'. A description with the justification of each technique and how the method contributes to the understanding of the phenomenon must be presented. Remember, it is necessary to provide enough description of each method to enable a reviewer with little knowledge of qualitative methods to understand how data will be collected and analysed. Give examples, suggest how the results will appear and what kind of information that each method used will produce. Add specifics of methods of model development, and list clearly all experiences that you, as an investigator, have had. Because of the nature of the qualitative proposal, the agency is funding you, an investigator with a good topic, rather than the proposal *per se*.

The ethical constraints of the project must be identified and discussed. Does the project address a sensitive topic? How will the project be explained to participants? Are they aware of their 'rights'? How will the anonymity of participants be protected? How will data be stored? Will data be used for subsequent projects?

Timeline

The timeline is a schedule or work plan for the completion of the research. The plan includes all the research tasks to be completed, a predicted length of time each task will take to complete and when it will be performed. This plan may be described as text but, because several tasks may be conducted concurrently, it is more frequently presented as a table or a line graph. An example of a timeline is presented in Appendix A.

One word of warning: when researchers prepare a timeline, they are often overly optimistic and do not allow for problems that invariably occur in research which causes delays. For example neophyte researchers do not allow realistically for the time it takes to enter an organization and begin to feel comfortable enough to start data collection. It takes time for trust to be developed and to locate appropriate participants. There may be delays with the interview process, and transcribing tapes and analysing data is an extraordinary time-consuming process. Even at the stage of writing, writer's block may paralyse a researcher. A rule of thumb is to estimate how long each task will take, and **triple** the time allowed. Such leeway is important because, if the researcher is hiring staff, enough funds must be requested for staff to allow for the completion of the project.

Budget

Again, when preparing a research budget, all research tasks must be predicted and costed, and then an additional allowance for unpredictable disasters, delays and rising costs added on to the initial estimated cost. Furthermore, because the qualitative researcher does not know and cannot predict how many participants will be interviewed until saturation is reached, then the researcher must be generous in this estimation when predicting costs. Nevertheless, there are some 'rules of thumb' when preparing a budget. A reasonably fast typist (over 60 words per minute) with a clear, recorded interview and a transcriber with a foot pedal, will take four times the interview time to transcribe it. This means that a 45-minute interview will take a typist three hours' transcription time. However, if the participant has an accent, if the recording is not loud and clear, this time will be increased accordingly. Because the transcription cost increases with poor sound quality, then it is false economy to conduct the research without excellent tape recorders, quality tapes and an external microphone.

When preparing a budget, mentally walk through all stages of the project, listing all equipment, supplies and personnel that will be needed. Budgets are expected to be accurately costed, so select equipment and list it by make, model number and the actual price; and do not 'pad' or inflate the budget. When listing the cost of personnel, do not forget to add the cost of employee benefits. 'Supplies' includes such items as stationery, audiotapes and telephone calls. Estimate the cost of any travel that will be necessary for the interviewing of participants by selecting an average distance and multiplying it by the number of trips and cost per mile. If the project is to continue beyond one year, do not forget to add a 4% increase in budget for each year to allow for inflation. Lastly, as permitted by the agency, add the cost of attending a conference to present the results.

Finally, all items requested in the budget must be justified — in particular, requests for computing equipment. If the investigator already has access to a personal computer, justify why a second must be purchased, why new software is needed and so forth. If equipment is already available for the project, list what is available and the location of the equipment. In this way the agency knows that the work will be accomplished within the requested budget.

Appendices

Appendices consist of documents that are necessary to support the application. Often these are documents such as a copy of the informed consent form, a letter of ethical approval from the Institutional Review Board (IRB), letters indicating approval for the researcher to conduct the research at a particular institution, letters of agreement from consultants, letters of support attesting to the quality of the investigator's work, curricula vitae of the principal investigator and other key staff and, finally, if possible, previous publications authored by the investigator of preliminary work or related work. Remember, when funding a proposal, the funding agency is making a 'leap of faith' in supporting a project, and, because with a qualitative project, even the investigator does not know how **good** the final product will be (or even what the results will look like), providing all possible information about oneself will assist the funding agency in making the decision to fund the proposed project.

Appendix A Informed consent form

The informed consent form serves two functions: it serves to provide a written explanation about the project that supplements the verbal information provided prior to the signing of this form (discussed in Chapter 4) and a written verification that the participant has been informed about the nature of the project, knows what will be involved in participating, understands the purposes of the project and any risks involved, has agreed to participate and understands that he or she may withdraw at any time without penalty.

Consent forms are always written in clear language that a lay person with the reading level of an eighth grade education may readily understand. The form must contain the name, address, positions and telephone numbers of the investigators, should the participant later wish to contact the investigator with a question. If the investigator is a student, then the name, address, and telephone number of the student's adviser is also listed. There are signature lines at the bottom of the form, and two copies of the form are signed: one for the participant and one for the researcher. Regulations vary regarding the disposition of the consent forms and the length of time from the completion of the project that they are stored: the US National Institutes of Health presently require that they be stored for seven years beyond the completion of a project; other institutions may only require one year. A typical consent form is presented in Figure 3.1.

Telephone consent

As the means for audiotaping telephone conversations improves, telephone interviews are becoming an increasingly common technique in qualitative

UNIVERSITY OF SMITHVILLE

Informed Consent Form

PROJECT TITLE: Becoming a Patient

INVESTIGATOR: J. A. Doe, PhD, Professor   Phone: 654-3210

The purpose of this research project is to increase nurses' understanding of patients' experiences when first admitted to hospital and the socialization into the patient role. Interviews will be conducted at least three times, and each interview will last approximately one hour. During these interviews questions will be asked regarding your feelings about being a patient. These tapes will not be shared with the ward staff, but the final report, containing anonymous quotations, will be available to all at the end of the study.

There may be no direct benefits to you as a participant of this study, but there may be changes in care to patients following the completion of this study.

THIS IS TO CERTIFY THAT I, _____ (print name) HEREBY agree to participate as a volunteer in the above named project.

I understand that there will be no health risks to me resulting from my participation in the research.

I hereby give permission to be interviewed and for these interviews to be tape recorded. I understand that, at the completion of the research, the tapes will be erased. I understand that the information may be published, but my name will not be associated with the research.

I understand that I am free to deny any answer to specific questions during the interviews. I also understand that I am free to withdraw my consent and terminate my participation at any time, without penalty.

I have been given the opportunity to ask whatever questions I desire, and all such questions have been answered to my satisfaction.

_____   _____   _____
Participant   Witness   Researcher

                                                                _____
                                                                Date

Figure 3.1 Informed consent form

research. However, with telephone interviews the researcher does not meet the participant face to face, and this poses special problems in verifying that all the conditions of informed consent presented above were met.

Tape-recorded consent provides an alternative. The researcher prepares an explanation of the project in listener-friendly language, with questions that are answered by the participant to indicate consent. This consent portion is not recorded on the interview tape, but is recorded on a special tape kept solely for the purpose of recording consents. Some review committees may also require that a written information sheet, explaining the topic and listing the title of the project and the investigator's name and contact address, also be mailed to the participant, for the participant's information.

The procedure for obtaining telephone consent is as follows:

1. Initial contact with the participant is made. The study is explained briefly. The participant is informed about the purpose of the study, the length of the interview and the fact that it will be tape-recorded. The participant is requested to choose a private place to receive the interview phone call and, if possible, to select a line on which a 'call interrupt' service is not used. If the participant is willing, an appointment for the interview is arranged.
2. The investigator sets up the recording equipment on the telephone line, with the 'consent tape' in the tape recorder and the blank interview tape close by.
3. The investigator phones the participant, and then, after checking that the participant is ready for the interview and remembers that their conversation will be taped, **turns on the tape recorder**. The researcher explains that it is required that the participant provides formal consent to participate in the study and that an explanation of the study will be read to him/her. A recording is made of the consent statement being read and followed by the participant's responses.
4. The participant is then asked to wait while the researcher sets up for the interview; the researcher quickly removes the consent tape and replaces it with the blank interview tape. As all of the consents for a single study may be recorded on one tape, remember not to rewind the consent tape because, when recording the next consent, you will be recording over the first consent. Because the consent tape has a record of participants' names, store the consent tape in a locked cabinet.

Appendix B Verification of ethical approval
Institutions generally require that all research involving human subjects be approved by their Institutional Review Board or ethics review committee. Generally, if the researcher is not investigating a sensitive topic, such as an illegal behaviour, qualitative research is considered to be minimal risk and therefore receives expedited review. The important point is that it must be reviewed and receive clearance before the investigator may proceed, and the

letter from the chair of the review committee is verification that the study has been approved. Note that this review is for the protection of human subjects, not for scientific merit. Scientific merit is the responsibility of the investigator and is ensured (if the investigator is a student) by the student's supervisory committee, by the funding agency and, finally, by the review process that precedes publication. Such evaluation of the proposal includes the 'worth' or the potential of the topic to advance knowledge, methodological rigour, and the research competence or ability of the investigator. It is important that these two reviews are separated and that the purpose of each is clearly distinguished.

Consent to photograph or film
Consents to photograph (including videotaping) usually include additional statements in the consent form. This must include a statement that the participant understands that she/he will not receive any remuneration for the photograph and gives up all rights to the photography. The use of the photograph or film is also made explicit: will the photography/film be used entirely for research purposes, or will some or all of the photograph/film be shown publicly? What is the nature of the public release — at research conferences, for educational purposes, for general viewing, as on public television, or as a press release? If the study is dependent on the data obtained from the films or photographs, it may be wise to make the consent in two parts: 1. consent for research purposes, and 2. consent for release/publication of the photograph or film, so that the latter consent for release will not result in the possibility of a participant refusing to participate in the study.

Appendix C Consultants' letters of consent to serve
One of the problems for the researcher embarking on his or her first qualitative project is to provide evidence to the granting agencies that demonstrates, despite the investigator's neophyte status, that the research will be of adequate quality to meet scientific standards and will be significant. One of the best ways to ensure this is to select consultants in the areas that the researcher feels lacking in experience. The role of the consultant may therefore range from guiding and advising the researcher throughout the project to negotiations for the consultant to take over and to 'do' the analysis for the researcher, equivalent to the quantitative researcher contracting out the analysis. Most granting agencies are more comfortable with the first arrangement, provided there is adequate time budgeted for the consultant to provide adequate and timely advice. The problem with the most extreme model in qualitative research, is that there is typically a reciprocal interaction between the data collection and analysis, with the insights for further data collection being derived from the ongoing analysis. This cannot occur if the data collection tasks are separated from the person doing the analysis. Furthermore, except for semi-structured interviews, the analysis continues concurrently with data collection and not as a separate activity after the collection of data. Most importantly, one of the

features that ensures excellence is that insights often arise from the intimate knowledge of data. This is not usually achieved simply by reading the transcripts — rather, the person conducting the analysis should listen to all the tapes. Hence little time is saved by the person responsible for the analysis — the most important part of the project — not conducting the interviews. (Special techniques for overcoming this problem with team research will be discussed in Chapter 5.)

Appendix D Research site: letters of access

In order to fund a proposal, the funding agency needs to know where the study will be conducted and that the particular institution has agreed that the research may be conducted within their organization. This requires two letters: one from the particular unit in which the data will be collected (for instance from the health nurse or supervisor) and one from the management or Board that governs the institution. Obtaining such permission requires, first, that the researcher informally approach the supervisor or head of the unit and obtain support, and then, second, formally approach the Board for permission. As the Board will require a copy of the proposal and details of the proposal are contingent on the research site, the process of entry negotiation often takes place over several months. This 'Catch 22' situation is often managed by the researcher approaching the head of the department informally and obtaining a provisional 'go ahead'. Then, the researcher writes details of data collection at that particular site into the proposal, obtains a letter of support from the departmental head and makes formal application for permission to conduct the research on site to the Board.

The use of a research site usually involves some reciprocation by the researcher; minimally, this involves giving the staff a copy of the research report. It may also involve public acknowledgment (and therefore disclosure) of the institution, and the wishes of the Board should be clarified at the time of entry. Similar reciprocal agreements should be made with the unit, with a presentation of the findings to staff at the end of the study and copies of any publications provided as soon as possible.

Appendix E Letters of support

Letters of support for the research are not always needed but may be of assistance in gaining entry in some cases, especially in international work. Letters of support are usually from esteemed and well-regarded colleagues who are willing to attest that the researcher is diligent, honourable and capable of conducting good work. For international work, they may also attest to the fact that the investigator is a student or a faculty member at a particular institution.

Appendix F Curricula vitae of principal investigator and other staff

The CV should minimally list the investigator's degrees, present position and employment history, grant record, awards, most recent and most significant presentations, and all publications. Often the format of the CV is specified by the granting agency and requested on a special form.

Appendix G Samples of publications
For qualitative application, sample publications are most important as they are the best indicators to the granting agency of how the final results of the present study may appear, and it is usual to submit about three. Often some members of the review panel will be new to qualitative inquiry, and it is these publications that will assist them to recognize the contribution that qualitative inquiry may offer.

EVALUATING PROPOSALS

When the proposal is completed, the wise researcher first reviews the proposal from the viewpoint of a reviewer and also asks several col'eagues to review the proposal from a reviewer's perspective. This pre-review is necessary to ensure: clarity, comprehensiveness, consistency and accuracy.

The first is for **clarity**. After reading the proposal ask, 'Do I know what the researcher is planning to do? Have all the steps in the research proposal been presented in a systematic and logical order? Is the proposal written so that it makes sense to a reviewer unfamiliar with qualitative methods, the research topic and the researcher's discipline?'

The second read is to ensure that the proposal is **comprehensive**. Ideally, the text should be detailed enough to counter any argument or query that could possibly be asked. Additionally, the proposal should be detailed enough so that someone who is unfamiliar with the methods knows and understands what the researcher is proposing. In reality, these expectations are not possible given the limitations on length that many guidelines list for submission; but to read the proposal with this perspective is important, for often gaps that can be covered with few words may be identified.

The third check is to ensure **consistency**, comparing each section of the proposal with every other. For instance if the research method calls for unstructured interviews, check that the use of unstructured interviews is justified in the literature review (for example is it explicitly stated that little is known about the topic?), that the broad introductory questions will get the information required, that the sample is appropriate and adequate, that the equipment for the recording and analysis of data has been requested, that adequate secretarial time has been requested for the transcription of the interviews and that plans for analysis of the interview match. Consistency between the body of the proposal and the budget is particularly important, with all of the equipment required to do the work either requested and justified, or stated, if it is already available.

The last preview check is for **accuracy**. Check again the agency's guidelines to make certain that all the requested information has been provided, that the type size is appropriate, that the margins are correct and that the pages are numbered properly. Check that all the budget figures tally correctly and that all the pages in all the copies are present.

A very useful study for the purposes of those preparing a grant was conducted by Cohen, Knafl and Dzurec (1993), in which they analysed the summary statements from proposal reviews returned to qualitative investigators. The strengths of those proposals receiving fundable priority scores were: had logical and clear aims or objectives; addressed an important topic; had a comprehensive literature review; built on previous work; provided a research design consistent with aims; justified the sample and sampling procedures; allowed for multiple interviews within a reasonable time-frame; provided clear and complete plans for analysis and for strong consultants. On the other hand, problem areas identified were the converse of the strengths, the most common of which were: an inadequate or unfocused literature review; problems with the description of the sample (unclear or poorly justified sample, an inappropriate sample and unjustified sample size); inadequate development of interview guide; inadequate plans for data analysis and inadequate attention for demographic variables or variables within the setting. While some of these problems may appear unjustified criticisms for a qualitative proposal, remember that the onus is on the investigator to provide justification to the review committee of all the nuances of qualitative design. Take nothing for granted.

SELECTING EQUIPMENT

Research equipment is an important investment, as the quality of the data is dependent on clear recordings. Lost data due to equipment failure may be disastrous. Furthermore, if equipment is complicated to operate, data may be lost due to human error. It seems that every investigator loses at least one taped interview due to human error — perhaps because he/she forgot to turn on the microphone, used batteries that 'died' mid-interview or incorrectly connected the equipment. These lessons are so painful that the mistakes are not made twice! In this section, the most common types of equipment required for qualitative research will be described, as well as common features to look for when selecting equipment.

When preparing the proposal, it is important to list the make, model number and cost of selected equipment, and justify its purchase. If the equipment is to be used in hospitals, check local regulations. Because of fire hazard, industrial quality equipment is usually required, and all equipment must be inspected and approved by the institution's engineering department prior to use.

Tape recorders and microphones should be selected with consideration for the purpose for which they will be used. Styles of tape recorders range from the microcassette recorder to the recorder that takes a full-size audio cassette. When making your selection, some features are particularly useful. First, the recorder must have a jack for an external microphone. If the recorder has a light that indicates when it is receiving the voice, that is also useful. Less useful are recorders that have a steady light that only indicates that the recorder is on, is recording and has an adequate power supply. A tape counter will enable the researcher to fast-forward to sections on the tape. An external jack to insert a foot pedal is an advantage because it will allow the researcher to listen to the tape, leaving hands free for making notes, and thus, if necessary, the recorder can also serve as a transcriber. The size of the recorder may be important, for it may be necessary to carry the recorder in the pocket of a lab coat. However, the most important feature is the recording time: the recorder must be capable of recording for at least 45 minutes on each side of a tape. Finally, the recorder should be sturdy enough not to fail in the field.

Microphones are available in a bewildering assortment of sizes and shapes. For research, a flat, 'credit card' style is preferable to one that looks like something a rock star might use, for the microphone may cause participant stage fright and interfere with data collection. Most microphones require a battery power source and therefore need to be turned on in order to record. The range and direction of the pickup is important. For example in a focus group situation, the microphone will require a different range to pick up the voices of the group than one used in a face-to-face interview. Therefore, obtain the advice of a technician when selecting this equipment.

A transcriber is important for efficient and accurate transcriptions of audiotapes. Earphones for the typist are essential to protect the confidentiality of the participants, and a foot pedal if the typist is to maintain a satisfactory typing speed.

The selection of a computer is in part a personal choice, depending on the type of computer the researcher is already using, and anticipated usage must be considered. For instance, is a laptop to take into the field essential or will a larger computer with video interface be needed? How much memory is needed and what size should the screen be?

Videotape equipment must be selected according to the needs of the study. For instance when working in a limited area, it is preferable to mount the cameras on the wall or ceiling of the room, with the cameras controlled outside the room to reduce reactivity to the video camera. However, if the patient is mobile, then a camera mounted on a tripod will be needed. All equipment must be set up and tested well ahead of time, to ensure that the quality of the recording is satisfactory. The quality of the sound, in particular, is difficult to maintain in the hospital setting because of the white noise from the ventilation system. Comply with the institution's regulations — for instance in North America, hospital regulations require that all equipment used in patient areas be of industrial quality and safety checked by the electrical engineering department prior to installation.

INFORMED CONSENT: SPECIAL CONSIDERATIONS

When coercion to participate in the research is low, 'implied consent' is frequently used. Consent may be implied, for example when the respondent receives the questionnaire in the mail, completes it, is assured of anonymity (and therefore does not sign it), and returns it by mail to the researcher. It may be assumed that the respondent consents to participate in the study by freely completing and returning the questionnaire. The alternative would be to put the questionnaire in the wastepaper basket.

Another example of implied consent is the confidential use of hospital records for research purposes. By consenting to admission and treatment in a research hospital, the patients are giving implied consent for their hospital records to be used for research purposes. However, such projects must be cleared through the institution's ethics review committee, and the researcher is expected to protect the confidentiality of the records, including the patients' identities.

When wishing to conduct research on 'special populations', such as prison inmates, hospitalized patients or school children, it is necessary to obtain several levels of consent. Firstly, permission must be obtained from the institution responsible for the individuals who will be participants in the study. The administrator or the ethical review committee will examine the proposal to determine that the health of those for whom they are responsible will not be jeopardized by the proposed research.

The next level of consent must be obtained from the legal guardian of patients (if the proposed subjects are mentally incompetent or if they are children). Finally, the individuals who will participate in the research must also give their own consent to participate. If the participant is a child and old enough to understand the procedures, then the child's **assent** must be obtained. In this case, verbal consent is adequate.

There are exceptions to obtaining parental consent, and such decisions will need to be made by an ethics committee. One example of this would be if the researcher wished to study adolescent pregnancy and informing the parents in the study also meant informing them of their daughter's pregnancy, which would be a violation of the adolescent's privacy. As the legal policy regarding this situation varies from region to region, it is recommended that the researcher seek advice regarding local laws.

ANTICIPATING DILEMMAS IN DATA COLLECTION

Qualitative research introduces special moral and ethical problems that are not usually encountered by other researchers during data collection. Perhaps because of the unstructured conversational tone of interviews and the intimate nature of the interview process, participants may tend to share other information — rather like a counselling session. With participant observation, in becoming a part of the setting, the researcher is exposed to all aspects of the environment. Even if those aspects from which the moral and ethical dilemmas arise are not a part of the research study, the researcher, by virtue of being present and being a witness, has a responsibility to the participants. The following example for discussion illustrates one dilemma arising from such situations.

> As a part of her thesis requirements, Joan chose to examine the supportive/therapeutic relationships among patients in a psychiatric ward. She had a great deal of difficulty getting access into the only psychiatric hospital in the city where she lived . (Actually, the process of approval took six and a half months of her second year.) Finally, she was permitted to observe and to conduct interviews in a 'less sick' ward.
>
> After two months she felt more relaxed in the setting and the staff and the patients began to trust her. Occasionally patients reported to Joan that staff members 'hated' and 'were mean' to them. Joan recorded these statements in her field-notes, but, as examining the staff-patient relationship was not included in her research question, she was careful to avoid such discussions during taped interviews. She noted in her field-notes that she thought certain patients were paranoid.
>
> One day, however, Joan arrived on the ward to find the place in an uproar. A patient accused a staff member of 'rough-handling' her. The patient had a large bruise on her back. The staff member denied the allegations. The patients appealed to Joan for help.

This example represents a typical dilemma in a fieldwork situation. In this case the subjects of Joan's study were in a powerless position, yet they perceived Joan (also in a powerless situation) as being more powerful and filling the role of advocate. Although Joan had conducted observations in the ward for two months, she had not observed any abusive behaviour of the staff towards the patients, and, due to the psychiatric illnesses experienced by the patients, it was possible that the allegations were not true. On the other hand, more than one patient had reported negative attitudes of the staff towards the patients.

Joan felt she had a lot to lose by 'taking sides'. She would lose more than a year of work, including the time taken to prepare a proposal, gain entry and start data collection. While presenting what she had been told by the patients would add credence to their complaints, it would also result in Joan having to withdraw from the setting. As she has no alternative research setting in her town, if she withdrew she would have to travel to another town or start again with another question, another proposal ... What should Joan do?

Estroff and Churchill (1984, p. 15) note that two of the most problematic situations for the researcher in a clinical setting are: 'getting caught between the patients and staff, and being privy to unethical and perhaps illegal conduct by staff'. They point out that in the clinical setting both the patients and the staff are the research subjects, regardless of the focus of the research question. Refusing to become involved in such a situation in order to maintain access to the research setting is indefensible, since it places the value of the research *per se* above the quality of life of the patient.

Joan is not in a position to 'know' if all, some or one member of the staff is involved in the present situation. One thing is clear: staff–patient relationships have deteriorated to a 'non-therapeutic' level. Therefore, one of Joan's goals must be to assist in the reconstruction of staff–patient relationships without taking sides. If Joan does have 'evidence' of staff maltreatment of patients, even if this evidence is in the form of patient reports, she is obligated to report these events. To remain silent and do nothing involves Joan in the abuse problem. A possible way to avoid these dilemmas is to anticipate the possibility of witnessing an undesirable event and to establish prior reporting arrangements with senior staff (e.g. the patient advocate or ombudsman), so that prearranged procedures may be followed should an unfortunate event occur. Having such channels identified will not prevent the conflict involved with such incidents, but it will set out an orderly, professional standard to be followed that will 'respect the rights and obligations of all interested parties' (Estroff and Churchill, 1984, p. 15).

PRINCIPLES

- While it is not possible to develop a rigid protocol for a qualitative proposal, the researcher must justify the methods used and explain **why** aspects of the proposal cannot be presented precisely.
- The primary objective of the qualitative proposal is to convince funding agencies and supervisory committees that the proposal is important, the topic worth investigating, that the methods are appropriate and the investigator is capable of conducting the study.
- The researcher must be familiar with the literature, yet not let the literature guide the investigation.
- Qualitative researchers do not let the proposal 'drive' the study.

- The proposal should be written to entice the audience and to conform to the constraints for the funding agency.
- Research takes at least three times longer than originally estimated. Plan the timeline accordingly.
- Do not pad the budget — make it realistically reflect costs.
- The investigator should request that colleagues review the proposal for consistency, comprehensives, clarity and accuracy before submitting it to the funding agency.
- Practise obtaining consent before beginning the study and anticipate ethical and moral dilemmas.

REFERENCES

Agar, M.H. (1980) *The Professional Stranger: An Informal Introduction to Ethnography*, Academic Press, New York.

Cohen, M.Z., Knafl, K. and Dzurec, L.C. (1993) Grant writing for qualitative research. *Image: Journal of Nursing Scholarship*, **25**, 151–6.

Estroff, S.E. and Churchill, L.R. (1984) Comment I (ethical dilemmas). *Anthropology Newsletter*, **25**(7), 15.

Glaser, B.G. (1978) *Theoretical Sensitivity*, The Sociology Press, Mill Valley, CA.

Van Gennep, A. (1967/92) The research topic: or, folklore without end, in *Qualitative Health Research*, (ed. J.M. Morse), Sage, Newbury Park, CA, pp. 65–8.

FURTHER READING

Marshall, C. and Rossman, G.B. (1989) *Designing Qualitative Research*, Sage, Newbury Park, CA.

Morse, J.M. (1991) On the evaluation of qualitative proposals [editorial]. *Qualitative Health Research*, **1**(2), 147–51.

Morse, J.M. (1993) Designing funded qualitative research, in *Handbook of Qualitative Methods*, (eds N. Denzin and Y. Lincoln), Sage, Newbury Park, CA, pp. 220–35.

Sandelowski, M., Davis, D.H. and Harris, B.G. (1989) Artful design: writing the proposal for research in the naturalist paradigm. *Research in Nursing and Health*, **12**, 77–84.

4 | Principles of doing research

Once the proposal is approved, and institutional approvals and funding have been obtained, the actual research can start. Beginning researchers (and even the more experienced embarking on a new project) report that starting is a very stressful time, and that knocking on the door of the first participant was the most difficult thing they had ever done. This difficulty may arise from the lack of structure in the qualitative research process, which leaves the researcher feeling that a lot could possibly go wrong (for example, that a prospective participant will refuse to enter the study). On the other hand, if participant observation is a part of the design, there is the awkwardness of not knowing 'what to do' or how to fit into the research setting.

There are several strategies that lead to the process of starting and give the new researcher confidence. The first is to role-play the consent procedure with colleagues. Practise explaining the study, answering their questions about the study, and obtaining their consent. This will do much to relieve anxiety in the first few days. A second strategy is to mentally walk through possible scenarios, in order to be best prepared for predictable events. For example, staff and clients will typically be asking, 'What are you researching?' Those asking this question do not expect a lengthy presentation but only a one-sentence reply. However, 'I'm not sure yet' will not do, as the researcher will likely lose credibility or the trust of the inquirer, who will immediately conclude that the researcher is either secretive or incompetent. On the other hand, the researcher's reply should not be so long that it will keep the person from his/her work, nor so specific that it will change participant behaviour. In addition, it must be consistent with the explanation on the consent form. For example, when Morse was beginning to study comfort in the trauma room and told staff she was studying 'comfort', the staff responded with, 'Well, we don't have time for that — go somewhere else!' (Morse, 1992). But if the reply was, 'I'm studying the ways nurses help patients in agony endure and maintain control,' the staff considered that a legitimate, interesting and important topic. Thus, the researcher must prepare an answer — a one-liner — to be ready for this predictable question.

GAINING ENTRANCE

In the last chapter, the importance of selecting a study site and obtaining official permission to conduct research was discussed. However, many months may have passed since obtaining the initial permissions and being actually ready to enter the setting. In this interval, touch base now and then keep the personnel at the research site informed of your schedule and the progress you are making. This is truly important, for conditions at the site may change, and the features of interest to the researcher for selecting the site may be altered during this period. One example is a study planned to explore the effects of removal of restraints in a psychogeriatric setting. Morse approached a clinical site, obtained Nursing's preliminary approval to conduct the study, and left a copy of the proposal (which of course reviewed the literature on restraint use). Two months later, when she had received funding and the formal permissions to conduct the study, she returned to the unit to arrange a start date. She was stunned when the head nurse said, 'You know, that was such a good idea [about removing restraints], we went ahead and tried it.'

'Getting in' involves gaining, building and maintaining trust with the participants you wish to study. Kaufman (1994) discusses some of the dilemmas inherent in the process of getting in and notes that gaining and maintaining trust is both an initial and ongoing activity of the researcher. It is critical to learn about politics and conflicts within an institution. In a recent study of change in a hospital, one researcher initially found she was not trusted. The reason was that Administration had introduced the research, and the nurses neither liked nor trusted the senior nurses in the institution. It took much time and effort to overcome the initial barriers and gain participant trust.

As a means of entry into an organisation, Field (1983) was given permission to speak to all the public health nurses employed by an agency at a general meeting. The study was submitted to the agency for approval only after it was apparent that the nurses were interested in taking part in the research. When two clinics were selected for the study, further meetings were held with the staff to ensure that they were fully aware of the nature of the study before interviewing and observation were initiated.

BEGINNING DATA COLLECTION

In qualitative research, the researcher is the primary instrument for data collection, and the collection of quality data is not assured simply because consent for the study has been given. Over time, the effectiveness and the efficiency of data collection varies. Initially, data collection is inefficient, as researcher comprehension is low (Figure 4.1). The researcher will have to establish credibility within the setting that is to be studied. The researcher must acquire the skill of being present and being trusted, without being close to one

OBSERVER

Comprehension	Low: confusion and bewilderment	Moderate	Maximal	Poor (perception distorted)
Effectiveness	Low	Moderate	Maximal	Low
Objectivity	Disturbed (stress)	Maximal	Moderate	Lost
Data collection	Unfocused — collect hard data (e.g. census)	Efficient and focused	Efficient and focused	Seek missing information only

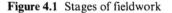

Data analysis		Begins	Directs inquiry	
	Stage I: Negotiating entry	Stage II: Selecting participants	Stage III: Acceptance/ cooperation in setting	Stage IV: Withdrawal from setting

Time

Figure 4.1 Stages of fieldwork

particular person, affiliated with one particular subgroup, or taking sides. It is necessary to 'be like' the groups one is studying, yet paradoxically, to 'keep one's distance'. There is a long-standing debate in the literature as to whether or not male anthropologists can obtain accurate information on women's cultural activities in pre-industrialised society (Gregory, 1984), and whether women anthropologists can converse openly with men in American Indian cultures (Wax, 1971, p. 46) or obtain information on men's activities (Bowen, 1964; Golde, 1970). Similarly, it may be questioned whether nurse-researchers can get accurate information on the perceptions of patients if they are seen to be a part of the nursing staff. Patients may perceive the nurse-researcher to be 'one of them' and worry about ramifications if they report negative instances of care. The way in which researchers present themselves to a group may therefore be crucial to subsequent acceptance, the quality of the data and the validity of the study.

Establishing rapport

It is essential that the researcher fit into the setting with minimal disruption. The selection of dress may also influence one's acceptance, as will observing rules of etiquette such as the correct form of address ('What would you like me to call you?'). In general, it is important to fit in with the group norms. Attention to detail at this stage will facilitate access to sound information as the study progresses. While it is important to establish commonalties with the group, at the same time there is a need to keep a low profile. While the researcher must establish credibility, to try to be better than the group will not be helpful in gaining their acceptance.

One critical factor in the initial stage of gaining entry is to demonstrate political, institutional and personal neutrality in the situation (Kaufman, 1994). It may be necessary to find a leader or informal leader who will introduce you to the group. Lipson (1991) noted that her experience of having a caesarean section helped to establish her credibility with her participants and opened up group communication. As a Caucasian female studying Black males, Kaufman (1994) describes how as an outsider she had to demonstrate that she was really interested in the group members as individuals and not just as subjects for study. She also points out the need to follow the rules and customs of the group; in her case this meant signing in on the sheet used by members to document their attendance at a day care programme.

As mentioned in Chapter 3, when entering the field, the participants will want to know details of the methodology and the purpose of the study. It is important not to conceal information, but it is necessary to keep explanations simple, brief and to the point. It is also important to indicate the type of information that will be used in the final document. It may be necessary to tell the participants that the content will evolve as the study progresses.

There is also some debate about the amount of 'distance' one should have from the setting, in order to collect and analyse data adequately. It is generally agreed that nurses should not conduct qualitative studies in the unit in which they are working. First, the confusion of roles as an employee and as a researcher and if information is 'research data' or 'patient information to be charted' can cause immense dilemmas that may result in misunderstandings, the violation of promises of confidentiality in the researcher role, or the withholding of information as a staff member. Of greatest concern is that data analysis may be impeded because of the researcher's familiarity with the setting. Nurses may not record data on some behaviour or other because the behaviour may be normative and therefore beyond awareness.

If the researcher feels there is no choice but to collect data in the work setting, there are a few precautions that may prevent problems. The first is to be aware of role conflict. It is difficult to work and to collect data at the same time, so ensure that all staff and patients know when you are in your researcher role and when you are a staff member. This includes making staff aware that, unless it is an emergency, as a researcher you are not available to assist with care. The second is to define the research question so that it refocuses one from one's usual perspective. For instance, if the usual role for the researcher is a nurse in the ICU, an important and valid topic might be to investigate the role of social support in the ICU (Hupcey and Morse, in review), so that, rather than viewing the setting as a nurse, the researcher is refocusing on the role of relatives and patients. However, maintaining confidentiality means withholding all information that is acquired, even including examples of excellent care. The golden rule is that no feedback is given to staff until the study is completed, and then feedback is given as a part of the analysis, with identities of participants concealed.

It is helpful to remove oneself from one's immediate work setting, if possible, as this action will assist in identifying implicit rules and rituals from the immediate setting. For example, in the previously mentioned 'Gift-giving' study (Morse 1991/92), eight research assistants (all graduate nursing students) assisted with the data collection. These assistants were assigned to collect data with nurses who were from a different speciality. For example, the graduate assistant with the speciality in ICU and cardiac care was assigned to psychiatry, the gerontology nurse to obstetrics, the psychiatric nurse to gerontology, and so forth. Using this method of assignment, the research assistants were able to learn about themselves as well as nursing, and this resulted in some lively debates. For instance, when discussing patient gratitude, the research assistant from ICU collecting data in psychiatry observed that 'psyche nurses do not think a patient's smile is a gift! They analyse it! They think, "Why did that patient smile at me? What does that patient want?" ' and laughed, much to the indignation of the psyche nurse, who felt compelled to explain about manipulative patients.

Try not to make unrealistic promises. It is not wise to share field-notes or give early feedback. Making participants aware of early findings may result in self-consciousness and behavioural change which could jeopardize the findings. Clarify the role: determine whether or not the researcher will become involved with nursing care and ensure this decision is communicated to all staff. It will be necessary to make clear both the extent and limits of any involvement, and this is a point the researcher will have to reinforce with the nurses over the course of the study.

The first contact is hard because the researcher is an outsider, a stranger to the group. The researcher must be able to accept the laughter of others when a mistake in etiquette is made and be alert to behaviours that to the researcher are suitable but which may be regarded as insulting to the group. As noted by Wax (1971, p. 370):

> The person who cannot abide feeling awkward or out of place, who feels crushed whenever he makes a mistake — embarrassing or otherwise — who is psychologically unable to endure being, and being treated like, a fool, not only for a day or a week but for months on end, ought to think twice before he decides to become a participant observer.

Despite the difficulty of these early contacts, once the researcher becomes familiar with the norms and values in the setting, things will certainly improve.

When observations are being undertaken, it may be useful to spend a week in the study area prior to the commencement of formal data gathering. This period can be used to get the participants acclimatized to the researcher's observations and use of tape recorders or video cameras in the setting. During this period the researcher should engage in all activities planned for the data collection period. The researcher must become familiar with the conversational patterns and normal behaviour of the participants during this period. The organisation of the group and the social interaction patterns within the group, as well as the informal leaders, should be identified. This period is critical because the observer seeks acceptance from the participants and establishes the research role.

There are some steps that can be taken to reduce the initial awkwardness of entering a group. The first step is to have an insider, that is, a group member, introduce the researcher personally to the group. Do not expect the first weeks to be productive. The initial period is used to get to know the participants while at the same time they are getting to know the researcher. Consider this phase as the time in which the feasibility of the study is being tested. Then, because it has already been acknowledged that this is a trial or practice period, mistakes are less embarrassing.

Wax (1971) notes that when entering a group, it is important to initially align oneself with those working in the lowest positions in the hierarchy. When entering a ward setting, this means first gaining the trust of the nurse aides and the orderlies, then the student nurses, the staff nurses, and, finally, the charge nurse. It is not possible to reverse this order and still be successful in gaining the trust of the whole group. People of lower status are suspicious of those who are 'close' to those who have power over them, and will be concerned that the researcher is providing the superiors with information.

It is useful to restrict one's inquiry to asking general questions in the first few days. Avoid topics that seem to cause discomfort or controversy to the participants. Above all, listen and learn the language and the values of the group. It is difficult to remember what everyone is saying when first entering a group. Do not try, otherwise panic will result. Rather, try to get a feeling for what is happening and use the time to become accustomed to the setting.

During these first days in the field, observe the organisational and power structure. Make notes on the setting and organisation at this stage. Who are the formal leaders? Who are the informal leaders? Who are likely to be key participants? For example, the researcher may be studying nurses, but the unit clerk may provide critical insights which would not be gathered from the nurses themselves. During this period in the field act like a sponge, absorbing all the information possible. When some grasp of the information is reached, then start to filter the data that has been absorbed.

The situational context of a setting has been described in different ways: environment or setting, ambience, or the immediate aspects of a situation. Miles and Huberman (1994) believe context to be the immediate relevant aspects of a situation, such as a person's physical location, their relationships with other people, and the relevant aspects of a social situation in which they function. Initially the researcher may not know what constitutes important aspects of context in a particular situation and therefore should make notes on everything, even if it does not appear useful and relevant at the time. In this way a more accurate picture of the context for the research will be obtained. Failure to record the obvious may lead to it being ignored or omitted, a problem to which the researcher must always be alert when undertaking qualitative studies.

Finding space

When a researcher enters the area where the study is to be conducted, it is necessary to find a space in which to work, in order to complete field-notes or diary entries throughout the day. Therefore, when negotiating entry also negotiate space for writing and interviewing. In ideal situations the researcher may be provided with an office with a desk and even with a locked file, but it is more likely the space will be a cramped corner in a storage room. The key factor is that the researcher needs space to write, undisturbed, so that field-notes can be completed reasonably close to an event's occurrence.

If there is no chance for the researcher to have a private assigned space, it will be necessary to negotiate shared space or find an unused corner in which to withdraw. A space that the researcher can use is essential if accuracy of data is to be maintained. If interviewing clients in their own home, it may be necessary to write or to dictate field-notes in one's car. Dictated field-notes should be transcribed within a reasonable period of time. Some researchers will want to type dictated notes straight into the computer. It is critical, however, to check one's field-notes for completeness before the observed event has become distorted by time.

While it is important to be accepted as part of the group, the researcher must avoid becoming too friendly with individual members. If friendships develop, there is a risk that the researcher and participant will lose sight of the purpose of the research. Confidences may be exchanged that can unwittingly become unethical in terms of the research, and this is how the researcher can lose objectivity and become caught in a bind of conflicting loyalties and interests.

Despite this warning, the potential for remaining detached and uninvolved is not always possible. Watson, Irwin and Michalske (1991) describe their experience in a longitudinal study that took place over a five year time span. They reported that in this longitudinal study bonds of friendship and concern developed and conversely, on occasion, there would be animosity observed.

Such feelings mitigate against complete neutrality and Watson *et al.* argue that a 'discriminating empathy' can enhance but need not interfere with an unbiased report. If such relationships develop, it will be important for the researcher to keep track of their feelings and emotions and to examine the effects of these on data interpretation.

Another concern is whether or not the observer will disrupt care. It is sometimes useful to prepare for data collection by entering the setting and identifying ways in which data can be collected which are not intrusive to the nurse and client. For example, Kratz (1975) found that note-taking resulted in a breakdown of the relationships she had established with her nurse participants. She decided that she would have to record notes after the interviews if she was to retain rapport with the participants. The researcher must be sensitive and responsive to the problems of the participants. If the researcher's schedule can be fitted around the nurses' schedules, the likelihood of being accepted will increase. Often it improves the quality of the interviews if they are conducted when the nurse is off duty, in the nurse's own time. This means that the nurse is free to concentrate on the interview without worrying about the amount of work to be completed before the end of the shift.

A frequent problem that is voiced at the outset of a study relates to the researcher's use of findings. In order to obtain ethical clearance, the purpose of the study and the mode of data presentation will have been identified. This information will also need to be shared with the participants. If data are being collected by a research team, inform the participants who will have access to the raw data and how the confidentiality of the information provided will be maintained.

Participants may wonder why *they* have been invited to participate in the study. The interest of nurse-researchers will probably be in studying nursing problems or care-giving with the end goal of improving care. It is important, therefore, to inform participants of this goal and to make it clear that while they may not directly benefit from the study, it is hoped that other nurses and/or patients will benefit in the future. Clarify the observer's role prior to entering the setting, and ensure that all staff are aware that the researcher is not there to assist with care or to evaluate staff performance.

In interview studies, the researchers may work with individuals rather than with groups, but the same process is needed to establish trust. In the case of studies of documents, the archivists will need to assure themselves of the researcher's trustworthiness and the purpose of the study before access to documents is granted.

Remember, small courtesies may make the difference between being accepted or merely tolerated by the host unit. The researcher is the guest, and the researcher must reciprocate. Bringing some food for coffee breaks helps — and often it takes a lot of doughnuts to get good data.

PRINCIPLES OF DATA COLLECTION

Data collection can be an intense experience, especially if the topic that one has chosen (and nurses often do this) has to do with the illness experience or other stressful human experiences. The stories that the qualitative researcher obtains in interviews will be stories of intense suffering, social injustices or other things that will shock the researcher. Data collection can become a time of intense emotional strain, with the participants' stories haunting the researcher so that the researcher loses sleep and becomes totally preoccupied with the research process. For this reason, it is important to pace data collection very carefully. Conducting interviews may be so extraordinarily psychologically draining and exhausting that not more than one or two should be conducted a day. It is important to develop a relationship with one's advisor or co-researcher, so that one may vent and debrief the feelings of distress arising from the study. It is important to take breaks from data collection, to exercise and engage in other activities.

Another hazard of becoming too close to participants is that the researcher may suffer with the participants. This involvement has the dual hazard of both interfering with the research process and overwhelming the researcher to such an extent that the researcher can no longer view the data analytically. It is important not to get involved and solve participants' problems. If participants are clearly in need of some assistance, then advise them where they can get this help. Exceptions to this golden rule are situations in which the researcher is legally obligated to interfere — such as with cases of suspected child abuse.

In qualitative research, data collection is a process in which the researcher learns about the research topic as the study progresses. Thus, there is a lack of standardisation in data collection techniques, and these change as the study proceeds. However, when the researcher is a neophyte, the lack of standardisation in data collection also occurs because the researcher is learning how to observe or conduct interviews, becoming more adept at interviewing as the study progresses. This is not necessarily a limitation of the study, but it may mean that the beginning researcher must collect more data perhaps than an experienced researcher.

With all qualitative methods but semi-structured interviews, there is simultaneous collection and analysis of data. This means that interviews are transcribed and analysed as soon as possible after the interview, and preferably before a second interview is conducted with the same participants. The interaction between data collection and data analysis is critical, for the analysis guides the data collection and the nature of subsequent interviews. A common problem with young investigators is that they become so busy trying to conduct 'good' interviews that they neglect to transcribe and analyse the interviews, and the study quickly becomes out of control as data piles up. Qualitative research is always a thoughtful, cognitive and deliberate endeavour, and the strength of qualitative work is in the analysis.

When conducting a participant observation, nervousness and feeling ill at ease often interferes with data collection. It is recommended that the researcher initially finds 'busy tasks' to alleviate some of this anxiety. Such tasks as learning everyone's names and roles, mapping of the setting, and learning the routine, will help to put the researcher at ease and use this time productively. When new in a setting, some of the participants in the setting will be anxious to befriend the researcher. It is wise to respond cautiously to these overtures, as it is known that those marginal members of the group are more likely to respond initially to new members entering the group. As we have mentioned, it is important to begin with the person with lower status than those who are supervisors or of higher status if one is to gain the trust of all members of the group. In addition to friendship, this role is also important for the process of data collection; that is, start interviewing in a setting by first interviewing those who are most junior.

PRINCIPLES OF SAMPLING

Two principles guide qualitative sampling: *appropriateness* and *adequacy*. Appropriateness is derived from the identification and utilisation of the participants who can best inform the research according to the theoretical requirements of the study. Because of the small sample size, the awkwardness in handling bulky qualitative data and cost of data collection in qualitative work, data collection must be effective and efficient. Drawing a participant randomly means that it is most likely that the participant selected may know nothing or very little of the topic — thus random selection is not only useless to the aims of qualitative research, but may be a source of invalidity. Theoretical sampling dictates that the researcher knows who best to invite to participate, based on the theoretical needs of the study and the knowledge of the participant.

The second principle is *adequacy*. This means that there is enough data to develop a full and rich description of the phenomenon — preferably that the stage of saturation has been reached – that is, that no new data will emerge by conducting further interviews, and that all negative cases have been investigated. Without meeting the criteria of appropriateness and adequacy, qualitative results are thin and the reliability and validity of the studies are possibly threatened (Morse, 1986).

However, there are some situations in which the researcher cannot determine which participants would be appropriate. The researcher may be using a volunteer sample in which potential participants are invited to contact the researcher. In this case the researcher should use *secondary selection* for sampling (Morse, 1989/1991), in which the researcher goes ahead and conducts the interview. However, if it eventuates that the participant does not have the information required or does not have the qualities of a good interviewee, then the researcher does not include the interview in the analysis. The interview is not transcribed or analysed but, rather, set aside. Nevertheless, the interview is not erased but stored, should further theoretical development of the researcher's project later reveal that the interview was pertinent after all to the research goals.

Selecting participants

Depending on the research question, participants may be obtained either from the community or from informal or formal group settings. If, for example, the researcher is examining breast-feeding practices, mothers who are nursing infants may be solicited from the community by requesting referrals from community health clinics or by using advertising methods to request volunteers. Even though some of these participants have volunteered to participate in the study, some will be more receptive to the interviewer and more articulate than others, and therefore be better participants. The researcher may not use all participants equally. If the research is to be conducted in an organization or with an informal group, there are key people who have more insight into the norms and values of the institution than others. It is important to identify these people and to obtain information from them. The researcher must be careful, however, not to ignore quiet, less verbally expressive individuals since they may have a different perspective on the institution. It is often easier to start data gathering with the more extroverted participant.

Douglas (1976, pp. 213–15) observed that any setting has at least four types of people that may be useful to the ethnographer. The first he labels 'social gadflies'. These are well-liked, lively, but low-key people. They have the ability to mix and to talk to almost anyone in the group. The second type are the 'constant observers, or everyday life historians'. These people are frequently older, long-established members of the group, who enjoy recalling details from past events. Next, the 'everyday life philosophers' are people who think a great deal about a setting, can provide insights into what is going on, but are generally less vocal than the 'constant observers'. Finally, 'marginal people' are those who do not really belong in the group or who feel ambivalent about the group and are the most common type of person used as a participant. Because of their split loyalties, they are able to describe an inside view and they are often willing to divulge information to an outsider. However, as they are often not completely trusted by the group, aligning oneself with 'marginal people' may stigmatize the researcher and impede the development of trust with other group members.

A participant may be any person who is willing to talk to the researcher. Participants are the key to sound ethnographic research and may supply the majority of the information needed, or complement data provided through observation, interviews, chart analysis or other techniques. When talking with participants the aim of the researcher is to find the things that are important to them and their understanding of the subject being researched. Because a researcher cannot be in all places at all times, the participant helps fill in gaps in the data and acts as a culture broker explaining the cultural rules, values, and norms within that setting.

Nevertheless, the participant may know only a part of the total social situation. Thus the acquisition of several participants who represent different sectors of the group is important. The use of several participants also helps to verify information. In a study of nursing, for example, the view of the supervisor, the graduate nurse, the patient, the physician and the ancillary workers may all be needed to understand the complex culture of a hospital ward. Germain (1979) illustrates this complexity in her study of a cancer ward. To understand the nurses' behaviour it was necessary to understand the norms and values of the total system.

In a busy organization, important conversations may take place over coffee or lunch or, in the community health setting, in the car driving from one appointment to the next. The researcher must take advantage of all such opportunities, but it should be made clear to participants that information obtained in these situations will be included in the study.

Once a relationship with a key participant has been established, the data acquisition will frequently snowball. The first participant will often introduce the researcher to other informed persons in the organization. The researcher should be careful, however, not to restrict participants only to those persons acquired in this way, otherwise the information obtained may be biased.

However, it is not usually possible to do in-depth interviews on all members in a setting. As stated previously, key participants are selected according to their role and knowledge or insights into the setting and the type of relationship they have with others in the setting. Another criterion for selection is the amount of rapport and trust potential participants have developed with the researcher and their willingness to participate in the research. If a key participant is not receptive to the researcher or to the project, then interviews with that person will be shallow and perhaps invalid as the participant will not disclose true feelings and may give only partial information on the topic. If the researcher does not have any choice and considers it essential to interview that person, then it is advisable for the researcher to take time and wait until a relationship develops before interviewing that person.

Thus it is important to note that the process of selecting participants in qualitative research is not done randomly. Selecting participants by statistical chance may severely affect the quality of the data because the participant selected by chance may not be co-operative nor be the best informed on the topic. However, by using such a subjective method to select participants to interview, it becomes important to constantly verify information obtained with secondary participants. Depending on the research topic, secondary informants may be all other persons within the same setting, or people in similar situations in other settings. In the first case, interviews with secondary informants may be more structured but still open-ended, so that the questions do not 'lead' the participant. In the second case, where the key informants are anonymous, the researcher may be more direct in verifying data or confirming the researcher's hunches. For example, when studying weaning practices, the researcher may approach other mothers who are weaning and ask: 'Some mothers have told me that weaning a toddler is just a matter of discipline. What do you think?'

These techniques of sampling in qualitative research have been criticized by quantitative researchers because the non-random nature of subject selection limits generalizability. Remember, the purpose of qualitative research is to discover *meaning*, not to measure the distribution of attributes within a population (Morse, 1986). Thus, generalizability is not the goal when undertaking this type of study.

THE ONGOING NATURE OF CONSENT

Having obtained informed consent at the beginning of the study, the researcher must recognize that consent may be revoked at any time by the participant. For instance, if, in the middle of an interview, a participant says, 'Well, just between you and me...', s/he is probably implicitly withdrawing permission for the researcher to use that information in the study. If in doubt, check with participant to see if the information so obtained may be included.

Occasionally the project will start well and then the participant will change his/her mind about participating in the research. The participant may withdraw from the study and leave the researcher with an incomplete set of data, or the participant may choose to withdraw all information collected about him/her from the study. This is the participant's privilege.

Another aspect of participant consent, especially with participant observation, is the continual nature of data collection. Data collection does not stop when the tape recorder is turned off, and participants tend to forget this. Frequently, when the stage of trust is reached, participants will treat the researcher as a peer and may, as one example, share secrets. This requires frequent and gentle reminders from the researcher ('Remember the study...') and permission to include that data. If permission is denied, the information cannot be included and must be discarded.

DATA STORAGE

The storage of data at the research setting may be problematic, for the researcher may not have an office or a locker in which to secure data. It is wise, therefore, after conducting an interview, to keep the tape on your person; for example, in your lab coat pocket or in a 'fanny pack'. As soon as possible, take data to your office and secure it. Some researchers immediately duplicate tapes so if one should become accidentally erased (due, for example, to static electricity), a backup will be available.

Tapes must be labelled with the interview number and the participant number immediately after the recording. Please ensure, for reasons of preserving anonymity, there is no link between the participant's name (on the consent form) and the participant's number on the data itself.

When arranging for tapes to be transcribed, it is important to explain to the typist the confidential nature of the data that she will be typing and that she should not discuss the data with anyone other than the researcher. Instruct the typist not to type in names but rather to put a line in the text followed by a parenthesis noting the relationship of the person that is being spoken about. For example, if the participant is discussing the doctor, the typist will put in '_____ (physician)' and then the text. It is important that the typist be instructed to type every single word of the dialogue and not to summarize the discussion. Long pauses in the text may be indicated with dots (...) and expressions typed (for example, [laughs] or [crying]). Short pauses in the dialogue may be indicated by a long dash (—). Instruct the typist to indicate any conversation that she cannot understand with '%' symbols, so that gaps in the transcript are noted and can be completed later by the researcher. As soon as the interview is transcribed, the interview should be checked for accuracy by the person who conducted the interview, and the hard copy duplicated and filed.

WITHDRAWING FROM THE SETTING

As the researcher becomes more confident with data analysis and works more intensely on data analysis, data collection in the setting gradually ceases. Prepare the participants for the time that data collection will cease by reminding them that, for example, you will be there for one week more. Making such announcements and giving participants warning that data collection is ending usually results in the participants providing as much information as possible to ensure that researcher has the story straight.

However, it is not wise to close the door completely in case the researcher finds a gap during analysis and realizes that it is necessary to collect more data. Therefore, when withdrawing, make sure that you obtain permission to return to the setting should it be necessary.

On the completion of the study, the researcher has obligations to participants. If the researcher has promised to return to the setting to present findings, make sure that this is done. Report back by mailing each participant a summary of the study. In addition, when the study is published, ensure that the staff receive a reprint. One final word: note that we have assumed that the study will be published. Unless the researcher makes an effort to publish the findings, the research process is for naught. Sharing the findings with the scientific community is both essential for the progress of science and, in reality, a most important step that is often missed. Again, without publication, all the preceding efforts of the researcher and the participant count for nothing.

PRINCIPLES

- To ease the stress of getting started, entering a setting requires careful planning.
- Successful data collection involves gaining, building and maintaining trust with participants.
- As the researcher is the primary instrument for data collection, it is important to establish credibility with participants.
- The researcher must fit into the setting with minimal disruption and maintain political, institutional and personal neutrality in the situation.
- When conducting research in one's own setting, it is necessary to demarcate roles as a researcher and as an employee.
- Do not make unrealistic promises to participants and remain detached from the group.
- Remember, data collection and analysis should proceed simultaneously.
- Select participants who have direct knowledge of the phenomenon or who have particular knowledge about an aspect of the phenomenon.
- Sample events as well as participants.
- Consent is ongoing, not static.
- Effective data collection is exhausting; adequately space your interviews and observations.
- Check equipment in advance.
- Ensure you have a secure place to store data.
- Warn participants at least a week in advance that the study is drawing to a close.

REFERENCES

Bowen, E.S. (1964) *Return to Laughter,* Doubleday, New York.

Douglas, J.D. (1976) *Investigative Social Research: Individual and Team Research,* Sage Publications, London.

Field, P.A. (1983) An ethnography: four public health nurses' perspectives of nursing. *Journal of Advanced Nursing,* **8,** 3–12.

Germain, C. (1979) *The Cancer Unit: An Ethnography,* Nursing Resources, Wakefield, MA.

Golde, P. (ed.) (1970) *Women in the Field: Anthropological Experiences,* Aldine, Chicago.

Gregory, J.R. (1984) The myth of the male ethnographer and the woman's world. *Journal of the American Anthropological Association,* **86** (2), 316–27.

Hupcey, J. and Morse, J.M. (in press) Family and social support: application to the critically ill patient, *Journal of Family Nursing.*

Kaufman, K.S. (1994) The insider-outsider dilemma: field experience of a White researcher 'getting in' a poor Black community. *Nursing Research*, **43** (3), 179–83.

Kratz, C. (1975) Participant observation in dyadic and triadic situations. *International Journal of Nursing Studies*, **12** (3), 169–74.

Lipson, J. (1991) The use of self in ethnographic research, in *Qualitative Nursing Research: A Contemporary Dialogue*, rev. edn, (ed. J.M. Morse), Sage, Newbury Park, CA, pp. 73–89.

Miles, M.B. and Huberman, A.M. (1994) *Qualitative Data Analysis: An Expanded Sourcebook*, 2nd edn, Sage, Thousand Oaks, CA.

Morse, J.M. (1986) Qualitative research: issues in sampling, in *Nursing Research Methodology*, (ed. P.L. Chinn), Aspen, Rockville, MD, pp. 181–93.

Morse, J.M. (1989/1991) Strategies for sampling, in *Qualitative Nursing Research: A Contemporary Dialogue,* rev. edn, (ed. J.M. Morse), Sage, Newbury Park, CA, pp. 127–45.

Morse, J.M. (1991/92) The structure and function of gift-giving in the patient–nurse relationship, in *Qualitative Health Research*, (ed. J.M. Morse), Sage, Menlo Park, CA, pp. 236–56.

Morse, J.M. (1992) Comfort: the refocusing of nursing care. *Clinical Nursing Research,* **1**, 91–113.

Watson, L., Irwin, J. and Michalske, S. (1991) Researcher as friend: methods of the interviewer in a longitudinal study. *Qualitative Health Research*, **1**, 497–514.

Wax, R.H. (1971) *Doing Fieldwork: Warnings and Advice*, University of Chicago Press, Chicago.

FURTHER READING

Aquilar, J.L. (1981) Insider research: an ethnography of debate, in *Anthropologists at Home in North America: Methods and Issues in the Study of One's Own Society*, (ed. D.A. Messerschmidt), Cambridge University Press, Cambridge, pp. 15–28.

Denzin, N.K. and Lincoln, Y.S. (1994) Introduction: entering the field of qualitative research, in *Handbook of Qualitative Research* (eds N.K. Denzin and Y.S. Lincoln), Sage, Thousand Oaks, CA, pp. 1–17.

Field, P.A. (1991) Doing fieldwork in your own culture, in *Qualitative Nursing Research: A Contemporary Dialogue,* rev. edn, (ed. J.M. Morse), Sage, Newbury Park, CA, pp. 91–104.

Freilich, M. (ed.) (1977) *Marginal Natives at Work*, Schenkman, Cambridge, MA.

Hinds, P.H., Chaves, D.E. and Cypess, S.M. (1992) Context as a source of meaning and understanding, in *Qualitative Health Research*, (ed. J.M. Morse), Sage, Menlo Park, CA, pp. 3142–256.

Punch, M. (1986) *The Politics and Ethics of Fieldwork*, Sage, Beverly Hills, CA.

Reason, P. (ed.) (1988) *Human Inquiry in Action*, Sage, London.

Van Maanen, J. (1988) *Tales of the Field,* University of Chicago Press, Chicago.

5	# Principles of data collection

Qualitative research encompasses multiple data collection techniques. The major mode of data collection is generally interviewing, often combined with participant observation. Interviewing techniques vary in 'standardization' from unstructured interviews or narratives to semi-structured (i.e. open-ended) interview schedules. Occasionally, the research design may include other approaches to supplement the interview data, such as structured questionnaires or psychometric tests, life histories, diaries, personal collections (letters, photographs), official documents and so forth.

The quality of the research project relies heavily on the researcher's ability to obtain information. No matter what methods of data collection we use, to be successful, perseverance and sensitivity are critical. In this section, the techniques of conducting the unstructured interview, the semi-structured interview and participant observation will be discussed.

INTERVIEWS

Most students think of conducting an interview rather like being a talk show host. The talk show image is a researcher sitting with two or three interesting and chatty guests, leading discussions about important topics in a witty fashion. Unfortunately, this is exactly what a qualitative interview is **not**. A successful qualitative interview is more like an intimate and personal sharing of a confidence with a trusted friend. And the information given must be treated likewise, with respect.

How does one meet a stranger and move to such an intimate and trusted relationship quickly? Several things may assist with the process. First, let the participant choose the setting: they may choose to be interviewed in the researcher's office, in their own home, their workplace or in a public place, such as a coffee shop. Wherever they select, it should be private with little opportunity for interruption; that means, for example being alone and taking the phone off the hook. Sit at a small table, for it is more comfortable than sitting in easy or straight-back chairs, and the microphone may be placed on the table between you. Take biscuits or cakes to the participant's home or, if the interview is at the researcher's office, prepare tea or coffee. Begin with small talk, start the interview with the consent procedures and, as the participant is expecting to be asked questions, begin by asking the demographic information. Then, let the participant lead the interview — you will find they quite quickly stop, looking for clues from the researcher as their thoughts become internalized, and they focus on their story.

The advantage of giving the participant control over the interview situation is made clear in the article by Davis (1986/92) in which she describes using a questionnaire. In her study on menopause, she confused her participants — women of a Newfoundland village — by asking them to answer by selecting forced choices that did not meet their situation.

The unstructured interactive interview

The unstructured interview is used when the researcher knows very little about the topic, is learning about the topic as the interview progresses, and as she/he interviews subsequent participants. Basically, the researcher does not have a series of prepared questions to ask because she/he does not know what to ask or even where to start. Furthermore, because the researcher knows so little about what is going on, it is important that the participant be allowed to **tell their story** with minimal interruption, at least during the first interview. A good starting question may be, 'Tell me ...', and sometimes the researcher does not have to ask another question.

Sometimes, however, the participant will need direction and ask further details, such as 'Where shall I start?' The answer to such a question is to let the participant start wherever she/he wishes. For example a doctoral student was studying the bereavement of spouses whose husband or wife had died of Alzheimer's disease. When the first participant began by describing marriage and then life with his/her partner before the partner became ill, the student turned the tape recorder off until the story reached the point of interest, that is the time following the partner's death. But the next participant also began the story at the same point, and the next. The important message is that each of these participant spouses was telling the student the same thing, that is one could not understand what the bereavement process was like, unless one understood what the marriage was like when they were both well, and what the marriage was like when the spouse developed Alzheimer's. Luckily, by the third interview the student realized this, left the tape recorder on and collected all the data. But the important point is that the participants often know better than the researcher exactly **what is** and **what is not** relevant to the topic.

When conducting an unstructured interactive interview, it is the researcher's main technique to listen intently. Assume an active listening stance and, even though the tape recorder is running, follow the participant's story carefully. Encourage the speaker with nods and the occasional 'Mmmm' and 'I see', but, by and large, be non-committal. Do not interrupt, unless as a listener you become hopelessly confused and need to clarify, for example who is who. Remember, you are **not** a counsellor, and the Rogerian techniques, such as reflective listening responses (e.g. 'That made you feel angry?'), are inappropriate as they lead the participant.

Occasionally the participant will get to a 'critical juncture' in a story. They will come to a part in which, for instance they had to choose between A or B and proceed to relate all about A. Later, when the participant has apparently come to the end of his/her story, take them back to that particular point ('You told me about A, but what about B?') and obtain the rest of the story. A good interviewer keeps track of the story, and it is this activity that new interviewers find so exhausting.

Because the interviewer is essentially a listener, it is hard to obtain a 'bad' unstructured interview. Occasionally the interviewer will ask a question which will appear irrelevant to the participant. The participant will politely answer it and then go back to exactly where she/he was before the interruption. This is called a **loop**. If the interruption is serious, such as the telephone ringing and being answered, then the participant may forget what she/he was explaining. In this case the interviewer should just repeat the last few words of the last sentence (… and he said …), and the participant will remember and continue as if they had never been interrupted.

While telling their story, participants will relive their experiences, including the emotional responses. For this reason, if the research topic is stressful, it is important to be prepared for sadness or anger. Narratives 'bring it all back' and, although a participant will not tell you anything he or she does not want you to know, it is wise to be prepared for the tears and have a box of tissues handy. However, it is important to note that it is this resurgence of emotions that is one indicator of the validity of this technique. When teaching interview techniques, an interesting class exercise is to ask one of the students to tell the class how the student met his/her spouse or fiancé(e). Often there is a short story attached to such meetings that the student is willing to share. After the student has told the story, ask the class to describe his or her affect — invariably it will be one of glee and delight in the reminiscence.

Occasionally, the participant will want to tell the researcher something that is very stressful or anxiety producing but will 'back off' the topic or stop telling the story, only to approach it again a few minutes later and perhaps be able to tell the researcher about the event. This is also called a **loop**. When this occurs, it is better not to interrupt or to force the participant to tell what event she/he is working up to tell. It is important that the participant remain in control of the pacing of the interview, and requesting the participant to tell such a story before being ready may result in the participant becoming upset and refusing to continue with the interview.

Unstructured interactive interviews have another important characteristic:

participants invariably tell stories sequentially, starting from the beginning to the end. As mentioned later, this makes the interviews very important sources of information for grounded theory where it is important to understand the sequencing of events in order to delineate the process.

How does one determine a 'good interview'? Good interviews can be detected as soon as they are transcribed. The page appears as a solid block of text — or the uninterrupted text may go on for several pages. If the researcher is interrupting, the text appears broken. The problem with the researcher asking questions is that the participant does not 'get into' his or her story and, after several questions, will stop the narration and wait for the researcher to ask the next question. Remember that the researcher has not planned questions because she/he does not know what to ask, thus it is a threat to validity to move into the question-asking mode.

The last questions at any interview should be: 'Is there anything you would like to ask me?' and 'Is there anything else I should have asked you?' Often this is the beginning of the real interview, as these questions are so revealing.

At the end of the interview, explain to the participant that you will transcribe the recording and think about it. Ask whether, should you think of other questions, you might contact him/her again to ask further questions? By the time the interview has been analysed, several questions may have occurred to the researcher: write these down. The second interview may be a little more directed than the first, more resembling a semi-structured interview, so that the gaps in the interview may be filled and the murky areas clarified.

Review committees sometimes express concern that the interview process may be stressful to some participants. This is not generally the case, even though participants may become upset during the interview. They generally express appreciation that someone has **at last listened** to their story. One burn patient noted that this was the first time he had had the opportunity to 'tell it all', and this in itself is an opportunity for participants to put it all together. Norris (1991) interviewed mothers giving consent for their daughters' abortions. She noted that even though the mothers became quite upset during the interview, by the time they had finished the interview they were laughing, joking and making small talk. The interviews were cathartic experiences, providing these mothers with a forum for the release of distress that they could not even share with their husbands. The relief was so complete that when Norris tried to phone back for a second interview, they politely refused. These mothers had closed the emotional door, felt they had nothing further to add and wanted to get on with their lives. Thus, the qualitative interview may be a very therapeutic experience.

Sometimes granting agencies are not content with the researcher's argument for using an unstructured interview and want to know examples of possible questions in the proposal. Indulge them — but do not let these listed questions constrict the study. Rather, list them as examples of possible questions, and use them only in the rare event that the participant insists that the researcher lead by asking questions.

The semi-structured interview

The semi-structured interview is used when the researcher knows most of the questions to ask but cannot predict the answers. It is useful because this technique ensures that the researcher will obtain all information required (without forgetting a question), while at the same time permitting the participant freedom of responses and description to illustrate concepts. For example when learning about the experiences of breast-feeding mothers, Morse and Bottorff (1989a) were anxious to find out about mothers' experiences in managing employment while nursing. They knew that employed mothers may have problems with leaking breasts (Morse and Bottorff, 1989b) or with expressing (Morse and Bottorff, 1988/92), but could not use a forced-choice answer questionnaire, as they did not know **how** mothers managed. Therefore, a semi-structured questionnaire, with short question-stems (the first few words of an open-ended question) that served as prompts, was ideal for this situation.

Because the semi-structured questionnaire provides participants with the freedom to explain a situation in their own words, try to establish a conversational tone during the interview. Try to get the participant talking, telling stories describing the incidents, and ask for examples and stories. It is these stories that provide the rich descriptive context that makes qualitative research so valuable and the analysis so interesting and significant.

When preparing a semi-structured questionnaire, think through the situation carefully and prepare the questions in a logical, possibly chronological, order. Each question should only address one aspect of a topic (i.e. there should be no double-barrelled questions) because asking more than one question at a time tends to confuse the participant. An example is in Davis (1986/92, p. 160).

> A: To what extent do you have worries and problems about your work about the house? ... [and then gives forced choices]
> B: Which do you mean, dear? Worry or problems? You can have one without the other you know. Mable over in Crow Grove ...

If it is anticipated that additional information should be asked, prepare the questions with probes, or additional questions designed to elicit further information. The questions should elicit discussion and should not be close-ended (i.e. questions answered with a 'yes' or 'no').

When preparing a semi-structured questionnaire, sketch out the domain of the topic and list in sensible order everything that you want to know about the topic, then construct question stems for each question to cover the entire domain. Check each question to ensure that it is **not** a close-ended question and list suggested prompts (e.g. 'In what way ...?', 'Please explain ...' or 'Can you tell me about a time that happened …?'). Next, pretest the questionnaire by asking the questions of a trusted colleague and recording the session. As the colleague attempts to answer each question, ask him/her to think out loud, so that any confusion is recorded and the nature of the confusion is clear. Revise the questions as necessary and then pretest on possible participants. Transcribe these responses, and check the responses very carefully to ensure that information is being obtained that will provide useful and interesting answers to the study questions. Revise the question-stems (i.e. the interviewer's question) accordingly and, if necessary, rearrange the order of the questions so that they are in the most logical order for the participants to answer. Create additional questions to fill any gaps and do not begin the study until you are satisfied with the question-stems. Remember: the quality of the study relies on the quality of these questions.

PRINCIPLES OF INTERVIEW TECHNIQUES

While the quality of the questions is important, the quality of the interview relies equally on the qualities of the **interviewer**. This section will be a pragmatic listing of hints for a good interview, points to avoid for a bad interview and what to do if things are going badly.

Characteristics of good interviewers

Good interviewers listen. They listen carefully and thoughtfully and stay 'with' the participant. Good interviewers are calm and settled and pretend they have done this many times before, even if this is their first interview. However, if their nervousness cannot be concealed, good interviewers honestly admit they are beginners so that the participant will take pity and help them through by being an excellent interviewee. Good interviewers do not fidget but give the participant all of their attention. Good interviewers are always able to prompt if, for any reason, the participant is interrupted. When the participant says, 'Where was I …?', the good interviewer can readily supply the last three or four words.

Good interviewers do not rush the participant, but wait. If there is a silence, then the good interviewer is not uncomfortable, for these silences are important, perhaps indicating that the participant is realizing something for the first time and having an insight about a particular event. He or she will continue when ready. Even if the participant is ready to ask another question, the interview is paced, not rushed — this is not an interrogation. Good interviewers check each tape and every transcript to critique their own interview style, constantly trying to improve.

Good interviewers realize that the participant is learning from the interviewer. They realize that if they use a special word, for example then the participant will learn and follow, using that word several times in the next few sentences. Good interviewers avoid using 'professional talk' because they do not want the participant to sound like a professional. Therefore, excellent interviewers do not lead the participant and play a very passive role. They are supportive, pass the tissues if there are tears, and give an occasional, 'Mmmm'. Katharyn May (personal communication, 1989) noted that the best interviewers are 'people smart'. Good interviewers can intuitively fit in with their participants, comfortable at home in a kitchen or in a boardroom.

Poor interview techniques

Many of these poor techniques that interfere with the quality of the interview are the converse of those behaviours that result in a good interview. However, they are so important that it is worth discussing again.

Do not ask too many questions, for the participant will then expect the interviewer to lead the interview and all the advantages of the unstructured interactive interview will be lost, a factor which may threaten the validity of the study. Poor interviewers ask several questions at once, so that the participant becomes confused; poor interviewers ask closed questions, readily answered with a 'yes' or a 'no'. Poor interviewers summarize the participant's responses and this makes the participant feel self-conscious. Poor interviewers also frequently verify the participant's statements, making the participant think that the interviewer is stupid, hard of hearing or not really listening.

Poor interviewers are ready to correct incorrect information that the participant has. They do not wait until the end of the interview to discuss any misinformation. They dive straight in, teaching the participant all they know about a topic, so that, when the tape is transcribed, it was very clear that the 'interview' was a teaching session. A role change occurs with the participant asking the questions and the interviewer answering. Thus, keep any teaching to a tactful session after the meeting is over. If the participant asks a question, divert it, continue with the interview and answer it afterwards.

Poor interviewers are nervous and ask questions so rapidly that the participant feels as if engaged in an examination. The nervousness is contagious and the participant eventually does not want to talk for fear of giving a wrong answer. Poor interviewers become impatient and, instead of waiting to see the relevance of a particular story, they interrupt. They are poor listeners and do not focus on the participant, rather they gaze around the room in a bored fashion.

Managing disasters

The key to managing a disaster is to try to predict the problem and plan a course of action before it occurs. The worst scenario is receiving a suicide threat during an interview. Luckily, this is a very rare occurrence. So, what does one do? If the person states they are about to do harm to themselves, try to get as much detail as possible to determine the extent of the suicide plans. Then remind the participant that the consent form only provides confidentiality to the extent allowed by law, and that you are obligated to report this threat. Try to persuade the participant to come with you to the hospital or make the phone call in the participant's presence. Researchers are also obligated to report crimes, such as child abuse.

A more common disaster is losing an interview because the tape did not record, became tangled or was accidentally erased. As soon as it is realized that a tape is lost, the researcher should sit quietly in a dark room and reconstruct as much of the interview as possible, talking into a tape recorder. If necessary, the participant may consent to being interviewed again, but another person should conduct the interview on tape so that it may become a part of the data set. If the same researcher repeats an interview, one cannot answer 'yes' or 'no' if the participant asks, 'Did I tell you ... ?', because the researcher may not be able to recall if the participant told the story during the lost interview or this interview. Unfortunately, every project has one lost tape, and after that experience — for it is always the best interview that is lost — the researcher is very careful with recording equipment and the handling of tapes.

Common pitfalls in interviewing

Interruptions

Interruptions by others distract the participant so that thoughts are lost and time must be spent regaining the level of intimacy established prior to the interruption. The most common interrupter is the telephone. If the interview is being conducted in the participant's home, ask if you may unplug the phone or take the receiver off the hook so that the interview will not be disturbed.

Select a quiet place where the chance of being overheard is reduced to a minimum. This will assist in the development of rapport and trust with the participant. Often nurse-researchers do not have any choice regarding the place of the interview: the patient is confined to bed. If this is the case, inform the staff that for the next 45 minutes you wish to interview the patient, and place a 'do not disturb' sign on the door. Inquire when medications, treatments or visitors are due, so that these times may be avoided. If the patient is in a shared room, a separate private place to conduct the interview must be found.

Competing distractions

A high quality interview will require concentrated energy on the part of both the interviewer and the participant. If while interviewing, the interviewer is concerned about being late for the next appointment, or if the participant is trying to supervise children or keep up with a television programme, it is not possible to obtain a meaningful interview.

Stage fright

Stage fright is common to all research where interviews are used to obtain data, but within the qualitative framework it may be increased, not least because of the use of the tape recorder. An open-ended interview also tends to make the interviewer feel more vulnerable; the tightly structured interview schedule used in quantitative research seems to provide a greater sense of security for the interviewer.

Stage fright may be a problem for the interviewer and/or the participant. The interviewer may have difficulty, especially at first, in 'settling' in to the interview. It may be difficult to ask certain questions, even though these questions are on the topic that has been preselected for the interview. For example if the researcher is studying the menopause, cues of discomfort or embarrassment received from the person being interviewed may make the interviewer reluctant to ask questions on such intimate matters. On other occasions, when both the interviewer and participant are more comfortable, the interview will proceed smoothly.

The second type of 'stage fright' relates to the participant's concern about the use of a tape recorder. As soon as the tape recorder is placed on the table, the tone of the participant's voice may change and become artificial. Free exchange stops, and the participant suddenly 'doesn't know' or does not have anything to say. The participant may protest that 'my voice sounds awful on tape' or that 'I don't have anything to say worth recording'.

There are several strategies to overcome these barriers. The first is to place the tape recorder on the floor, out of sight, and use a small pencil, 'credit card' or lapel microphone to pick up the conversation. Then, as the interview proceeds, the participant 'forgets' about the tape recorder and the interaction quickly becomes normal.

A second strategy is to use telephone interviews. Ask the participants if they would prefer to be interviewed by telephone, making it clear that the conversation will be recorded. As people are used to speaking on the phone, it is easier for them to speak freely (see Chapter 3).

Occasionally the participant will sense a social distance between himself/herself and the researcher. For some, participating in research is a prestigious activity, yet the notion that a **scientist** is seeking information, asking and listening to what **they** have to say, may be intimidating. In these situations the interview moves slowly and the participant's answers are short and given reluctantly.

When the researcher senses this problem, the best strategy is to 'play dumb'. Ask more probing questions, and respond with surprise or 'You're kidding!' Wax (1971, p. 370) notes that the researcher must 'see himself as an educated and highly intelligent adult, and, simultaneously, as a ludicrous tenderfoot or *schlemiel* who knows less about what he is doing than a native child'. Therefore it is best to accept corrections from the participant as instructive, remembering that learning through laughter and ridicule is an 'ancient if painful method of pedagogy'.

Avoiding awkward questions

It is expected that, in the course of an interview, many questions will be asked that are not normally a part of polite conversation. For instance when studying childbirth or infant feeding, it may be necessary to ask about marital status or income level. The participant may feel caught in a bind, not wanting to respond, yet feeling impolite and unhelpful by refusing to answer.

Initially the interviewer should decide if the question is absolutely necessary, given the risks of asking. For example the participant may be offended by the question and refuse to continue with the interview. As many studies have examined the importance of a support system and the dearth of breast-feeding in lower socio-economic classes, a question may be theoretically justified in this breast-feeding example. Risks may be minimized by placing this question last.

Another strategy may be to ask the question in a way that will remove some of the potential embarrassment. Therefore, rather than asking, 'What is your marital status?', the interviewer could ask, 'How many people are living in your household?' The response will provide necessary information regarding the presence or absence of a partner, as well as other people who may provide assistance. Does it matter to the researcher whether or not a couple are married? Remember, the researcher is likely to be interested in **support**, rather than in legal status.

Obtaining information on level of income is more difficult. One method would be to write **ranges** of income on a card and ask the participant to identify the range into which the family income falls. As these questions may interfere with the interaction of the interview, if they can be left until last, this should be done.

Jumping

Frequently, interviewers ask questions in an apparently illogical order. For example when interviewing a mother on her breast-feeding experiences, the interviewer may ask about the baby's health at birth, then about the baby's present health. The interview may continue with the initial breast-feeding experiences and then the present breast-feeding experiences, the initial support systems and then the present support systems. While this order makes perfect sense to the interviewer (who has organized the questionnaire for ease of data analysis), this order will not necessarily make sense to the participant. If the mother is trying to explain to the interviewer that her breast-feeding experiences at birth, her present experiences, her initial experiences and her support systems are all interrelated, it may be very difficult for the mother to explain one aspect of the situation at a time. Therefore the interviewer must elicit the information from the participant's perspective at her own pace.

Usually, explaining the experience in chronological order makes most sense in the first interview. Ask the mother to describe breast-feeding experiences from the first time she nursed. In subsequent interviews, when the participant realizes that the interviewer understands the complete picture, comparative questions may be asked.

Frequently the participant is nervous and tries to give the interviewer too much information at once. This is evidenced by rapid speech and disjointed thought processes. Statements such as 'And before that ...' and 'Oh, that was when ...' will be indicative of this problem. Stop the interview and ask the participant to tell the story from the beginning. Assure the participant that she has plenty of time and that you will come back for another interview if the story is not finished.

Counselling

Nurses, in the course of their education, have a great deal of instruction in counselling techniques. They become expert at reflecting and summarizing during an interaction. They frequently use phrases such as 'Are you saying that ...' or 'It seems to me that ...'. The use of these techniques too early in the interview, or the overuse of these techniques, will inhibit the interview, especially if it is on a personal topic. It is easier for the participant to agree with the interviewer than to explain how it **really** is. Preliminary analysis invites premature closure of the topic and precludes in-depth inquiry.

These problems are easy to spot in the typed transcript. There is imbalance in the amount said by the interviewer and the participant. In a good interview, the interviewer's responses comprise a much smaller amount of text than the participant's, that is the bulk of the transcript is description, explanations and clarifications provided by the participant. The interviewer's role is in guiding the direction of the interview, probing, understanding and encouraging. Confirmation and summarization of information should be left until the end of the interview.

Presenting one's own perspective

This is also similar to counselling, teaching and correcting misinformation. When explaining a particular process or event, the participant will look for signs of acceptance or rejection by the interviewer and use these cues to judge whether to continue. For example many mothers reject breast-feeding because they feel that it 'really belongs in the barnyard' or is 'animal-like'. Yet these same mothers know that this perspective is not shared by health professionals, therefore they may hint at this belief to 'sound out' the interviewer. Frequently these 'feelers' are presented in the third person ('I know that some people think ...') or as a friend's belief. If the interviewer takes a position on this belief, for example by expressing ridicule or disagreement, then the mother will not disclose her true feelings to the interviewer. As the interviewer does not know what the participant really thinks about breast-feeding, the feelings of the interviewer should not be revealed, but rather should provide an accepting sounding board for the participant. Do not be trapped by the participant's 'What do you think ...?' responses.

Superficial interviews

We are the best evaluator of our own interviews. In an interview situation the researcher has the opportunity to assess the non-verbal cues, such as eye contact, facial expression and body posture. As the interview progresses, the interviewer also gets to 'know' the participant, to learn when the participant is uncomfortable answering a question and does not wish to pursue a certain topic, or when she/he is speaking freely.

Frequently interviews are 'shallow' because the interviewer moves the participant along too quickly. The participant does not get time to reflect and explain all aspects of a problem before the interviewer has asked the next question. Using silence, acknowledging with 'Hmmmm', and giving permission for the participant to continue are the best ways to increase the richness and depth of the data.

Rarely can 'rich' data be obtained from the first interview, therefore do not close the relationship with the participant at this time. Rather, ask if it is possible to return if any additional information is needed after the transcript has been reviewed. Interviewing is an exhausting procedure, and the interviewer frequently feels drained at the end of an interview. However, after analysing the tape, many questions and areas that need exploring become obvious, and the researcher may need to continue with the interview.

Secret information

When interviewing, the level of trust may develop between the researcher and the participant to the extent that participants pass on information labelled as 'secret'. For example they may state that this is 'Just between you and me ...' or 'Don't put this in your report, but ...'. Alternatively, participants may provide information that is later regretted. They will state, 'I shouldn't have told you that yesterday ...'. As the researcher's **first** responsibility is to the participant, the participant has the right to retract information or to request that the information not be used in the report, and the researcher must respect the participant's wishes. Violation of this code will result in loss of trust and may have extensive ramifications for the participant.

However, occasionally information is passed on to the researcher which the researcher feels is the key and is essential to understanding the other pieces in the puzzle. In this case, it is appropriate to recheck to see if the participant will reconsider his/her decision so that the information may be included. Occasionally, a method may be worked out so that the information can be included; if not, forget the information.

Use of an interpreter

The use of an interpreter 'slows' the interview as each statement must be repeated in the alternate language. This is frequently an advantage, as it gives the researcher more time to reflect on the previous responses and carefully prepare the next question. It also allows the researcher more time to observe the non-verbal cues of the participant, such as facial expression.

However, there are disadvantages. Firstly, the translator may not accurately translate the affective meaning and expression of the respondent. The translator, rather than providing verbatim responses, may summarize the content of the participant's statements. Secondly, if a semi-structured interview is being conducted, and many people are being interviewed, the translator may become bored with hearing the same answers. Rather than translating the answers, the translator may turn to the researcher and say, 'same as the others', instead of reporting the participant's response.

These problems may be overcome by carefully instructing the translators in the importance of giving complete answers and the correct intonation, and by using more than one translator to prevent boredom.

Minimizing the dross rate

During the interview, it is the interviewer's role to guide the interview and to keep the participant on topic. The amount of irrelevant information in an interview is known as the **dross rate**. The dross rate may be high if the participant is an elderly person who is inclined to wander off the topic, or if the researcher permits himself/herself to be tempted into listening to irrelevant stories or lacks the ability to focus the interview.

The best strategy for minimizing the dross rate is to prepare several open-ended questions before each interview. It is best to begin the first interview with a very broad question, such as 'Tell me about your experiences with juvenile diabetes, when did it begin?' This will enable the researcher to obtain a relatively complete picture of the participant's experiences. The second and subsequent interviews may be more focused on particular methods of coping or eliciting feelings about the situation.

WRITTEN METHODS OF DATA COLLECTION

The short-answer questionnaire

The short answer, open-ended questionnaire is an appropriate form of data collection to use when some of the dimensions of the construct are known and when it is necessary to use a written form of data collection, but all possible responses cannot be anticipated. For example an open-ended questionnaire would be appropriate in a situation where interviews may cause embarrassment, and this was the ideal method of collecting data on the adolescent's response to menarche (Doan and Morse, 1985). Previous researchers had reported that little information could be obtained using interview methods as the girls were reluctant to express their feelings openly and responded with embarrassed giggles.

The short-answer, open-ended questionnaire takes the form of a short question-stem and space — usually one or more blank lines for the respondent to answer the question. As this method of data collection provides some freedom for the responses to the question, these data are more likely to be meaningful and valid. However, the emic or the etic perspective may be obtained depending on the wording of the questions. Consider two similar examples:

(a) Health is
(b) Health, to me, is

Answers to the first question (a) are likely to resemble known definitions of health, such as the early World Health Organization definition, 'Health is the absence of disease and infirmity'; whereas the second question (b) will elicit an emic definition, such as 'Health is when you feel good, and somebody loves you'.

When constructing an open-ended short-answer questionnaire, it is also important to consider the expected length of the answers and whether a question will require, for example two lines or six. Respondents tend to write in two-thirds of the required space, whether there are two lines or six lines, and the more they write, the more information the researcher obtains. However, there is an upper limit. Too many lines are intimidating and make the questionnaire appear as if it will be too much work and take too much time to complete. The best solution is to pretest the questionnaire. Ask a number of people to complete the questionnaire and examine their answers very carefully to ensure that the type of information required to answer the study question is being obtained. Then ask the respondents to 'critique' the format of the questionnaire for friendliness and effectiveness. While questionnaires of this type are more difficult and time-consuming to code than forced-choice questionnaires, they are easier to analyse than an unstructured interactive interview. They have the advantage that the researcher can compare answers to the same questions, and can analyse content and quantify the number of responses in each category for each item.

The major disadvantage of this method is that the respondents must be literate and comfortable expressing their views in writing. The technique would be suitable for use with university students but less suitable for use with other groups. People who hesitate to write because they feel that they cannot spell or people who are unaccustomed to writing will be more likely to refuse to participate in the study; this biases the sample. When English is the participant's second language, although it may be spoken with relative ease, reading comprehension and writing ability in English may be more restricted.

OBSERVATIONAL TECHNIQUES

Observation adds breadth to research and provides answers to contextual questions which cannot be answered by interview alone. It is, however, time-consuming, and the necessity for observation must be clearly justified as it adds considerably to research costs. Using observation also raises the issue of informed consent: how do you obtain a consent from everyone you observe, or, conversely, is this necessary if you are looking at a cultural group in which some of the participants are peripheral to the main study but happen to interact with the main participants? An obsession with informed consent could end naturalistic research; yet covert observation, such as that carried out by Rosenhan (1973/92) in his study, 'On being sane in insane places', raises ethical issues regarding consent that are hard to justify in today's society.

In some settings, such as a hospital unit (or ward), it may be possible to use the concept of 'not refusing'. This would mean explaining the study widely and then requesting those who did not want to participate to return a signed 'decline to participate' form. This would still leave the researcher able to question as to whether everyone had the chance to respond negatively, but would enable the researcher to proceed in a setting where many peripheral individuals may be observed. The main participants, who would also be interviewed, would still be required to sign consents.

There are studies in which the researcher claims to use participant observation as the method for the study (Nystrom and Segesten, 1994; Weinholz, 1991) rather than as the data collection technique. In these instances, one needs to look carefully at the description of data collection and analysis. In both of the cited studies, the method appears to be that of a focused ethnography, with observations, interviews, field-notes, etc. being used for gathering data.

The classification of types of participant observation according to the degree of involvement that the researcher has in the setting, described by Gold (1958) and Pearsall (1965) still hold true today. The primary purpose of participant observation is to observe participants in as natural a setting as possible. The researcher wishes to obtain an accurate, detailed description of the setting. It is also essential to ensure that the setting is minimally disrupted or altered by the presence of the observer. The researcher selects the type of participant observation with these factors in mind.

Participant observation

Participant observation is the second most common approach to data gathering used in qualitative research. It is essential for data gathering in ethnography. It is also used as an approach to data gathering in grounded theory studies and in some studies which use ethnoscience as the analytic method.

Observations focus on the context and include the reactions of individuals in the social setting and the structural — functional aspects of the society being studied. Observation enables the researcher to view the society objectively and assists in the validation and interpretation of information provided by participants. It can also be used to obtain a picture of the world of the inhabitants in situations where participants in the culture have low verbal usage, for example in nursing homes. In one Swedish study (Nystrom and Segesten, 1994), participant observation was employed to study patient reaction in a nursing-home setting with a focus on the structure and function of the institution.

Observation requires sensitivity to both the facial expression and body language of participants. The way in which these are manifested may be culturally determined. For example in some cultures, avoidance of eye contact is considered polite. It is also crucial that the researcher has prior knowledge of the history and, where possible, the social background of the group before undertaking the participant observation phase of the study. The researcher also needs to have a talent for making social contact with others. It is critical that the observer facilitate the expression of meaning while avoiding imposing meaning on the situation. The final caution is that accurate observation takes time. The researcher is sampling events and situations that occur within the cultural setting, and this cannot be achieved in one or two days spent in the setting (Golander, 1987/92).

Types of participant observation

Complete participation

When conducting complete participation, the observer enters the setting as a member of the group and conceals the research role from the group. A nurse interested in observing behaviours in the emergency room would therefore obtain an assignment to that area and not disclose the intent to observe and conduct research to the rest of the emergency-room staff.

This type of observation presents the following problems. Firstly, the degree of concealment of the researcher's purpose is rarely defensible. That is it is a violation of ethical standards to enter a setting and observe in that setting without the knowledge and consent of the participants. Secondly, it is difficult to be immersed in a work role in a setting and to objectively observe at the same time. As a nurse, one must pay attention to the assigned tasks rather than the setting as a whole. Furthermore, it is difficult to find time to make field-notes and to conceal this activity from the others. Gold (1958) also notes that the researcher may become so preoccupied with concealing the researcher role that she/he may not perform convincingly in the work role. In addition, after a length of time in the setting, the researcher may 'go native', lose objectivity and completely adopt the work role, therefore biasing the results.

Participant-as-observer

In this method, the participants in the setting are aware of the researcher's purpose and dual roles. When entering the setting, the researcher usually negotiates work responsibilities with the staff and delineates a small proportion of time for the purpose of writing field-notes, observing or conducting formal interviews. This type of observation is suitable if the type of phenomena under study is not constantly present in the setting. For example the researcher may be interested in postoperative pain and wish to observe patients recovering from anaesthesia. The nurse may elect to assume a work role at times that patients are not available to be observed.

This type of observation has certain disadvantages. Conflict between the two roles may occur when the nurse tries to 'work two jobs at once'. For instance if the ward becomes busy, the researcher and the staff may feel that the nurse is obliged to assist with the nursing tasks rather than continue with the research tasks. This may be frustrating to the researcher, especially if the missed research opportunities are a 'rare' event. Ironically, the source of the ward's business is frequently the phenomena in which the researcher is most interested, and the difference in priorities may cause conflict on the ward. It is without question, however, that if there is a life-threatening event on the ward, the researcher's first responsibility is to the patient.

Observer-as-participant

This level of participant observation, with the majority of the researcher's time spent observing and interviewing and minimal participation in the work role, provides more freedom to do research with less conflict. The main disadvantage is that the researcher may be considered an 'outsider' by the staff and not be trusted or given access to the insider's perspective of the phenomena. On the other hand, this level of participation may be needed to establish the researcher's credibility in the setting.

Complete observer

In this role the researcher is passive, having no direct social interaction in the setting. The observer may use video cameras, one-way mirrors to remain separate from the setting, or sit quietly in the corner observing the setting as a 'fly on the wall'. This method has the disadvantage of not permitting the observer to interview, interject or clarify issues with the participants in the setting. Again, as with the complete participant, concealment behind one-way mirrors without the knowledge of the participants can rarely be justified.

Selecting a setting

The most frequent mistake that researchers make when doing participant observation is to select a setting in which they already work, or have previously worked, to conduct observations. This will create several problems which will prevent the collection of valid, reliable and meaningful data. Firstly, if the nurse has already established a role or niche in a unit, the staff have certain expectations of that nurse regarding contributions to work. Even negotiating a new role will not remove these expectations, as the staff consider that nurse to be an ally who will help or 'pitch in' if the need arises. Furthermore, as a 'doer' it is hard for the researcher to sit 'doing nothing' while the staff cannot keep up with the workload. Secondly, the nurse researcher will already be integrated into the group, that is she/he will be considered a 'native' by those in the setting and have unconsciously incorporated the values of the group to be studied. In this case, it is not possible to be an objective observer.

If the nurse has not been in the setting for some period of time prior to the research, this can be an advantage or a disadvantage. When the nurse re-enters the setting, the period of strangeness and non-comprehension will be reduced so that the nurse will be able to begin meaningful data collection more quickly. However, the period of objectivity before the researcher 'goes native' and has to withdraw from the setting will be shortened considerably. It is important to select a setting in which the researcher will be considered a stranger. This may mean changing hospitals to conduct the research.

Problems with participant observation

The major difficulty interfering with validity in participant observation is the change in behaviour in the setting when the observer is present. This change is reduced over time when the participants become used to the observer, feel less threatened, and trust increases. Paterson (1994) calls this 'emotional valence' and suggests that it is representative of the feeling that exists between the researcher and the participants during the data collection period. The degree of trust will determine the nature of the data provided by the participant to the researcher. Trust is not the sole barrier to the sharing of information, however; the sex or age of the participant may also influence the information which may be given to the researcher. Data gathered when one is initially observing a setting may be limited by what the participants are willing to share. As the time spent in the setting increases, the researcher-as-stranger may become the researcher-as-friend (Leininger, 1985). While data will become richer as the study period progresses, there is also an increased risk that the researcher will go native and begin to subscribe to the views of the participants, thus losing objectivity.

The researcher must retain the freedom to enter and leave the setting as desired. Do not agree on an appointment system to conduct observations, for this permits the scene to be 'set' for the arrival of the observer. For example one researcher was observing in a paediatric ward. She was welcome to make observations 'any time but bedtime'. The staff thought that observations at bedtime would be disturbing for the children. In actual fact, the children's behaviour at this time provided the richest data on separation anxiety.

One method used to verify observations and to overcome this problem is 'spot observation'. With this technique, the researcher randomly selects times to make observations and enters the setting unannounced at those times. Morse (1984), while studying mother–infant interaction in Fiji, used this method. She was interested in the spatial distance between mothers and their infants, and made her observations as she entered the household at each randomly selected time.

Unequal distribution of power between the researcher and the participant may be another cause for concern (Paterson, 1994). There is the risk that subordinates with lesser power than the researcher may wish to respond in a way that will please the researcher. In a study of nursing students' socialization into nursing (Campbell *et al.*, 1994), this problem was overcome by having research assistants conduct the interviews and make observations. However, one interviewer initially was inclined to contradict a respondent because she believed she knew how the responses should be made. It is critical to monitor assistants to ensure that such violations in data gathering do not occur. Adequate time in the field and the development of trust also assist in overcoming this problem.

Another major problem in participant observation, as mentioned in Chapter 3, is the witnessing of unethical behaviours which interfere with patient care. For example the researcher may observe the slapping of a child, the refusal to give a patient in pain an analgesic or a bedpan to a patient 'for the 56th time that day'. If the incident is life-threatening there is no question as to the action required. Patient safety is paramount and the researcher intervenes. However, there is a grey area where the researcher knows that if the incident is reported it will result in a role change, and the researcher will become a 'policeman' in the view of the patients and staff. If the researcher interferes by getting the bedpan, a role change will also occur that will result in a change in the data. No prescriptive advice can be given, for each case depends on individual circumstances. Perhaps discussing the situation with colleagues or requesting the counsel of the ethics committee will assist in resolving the dilemma.

FIELD-NOTES

As it is difficult to remember many details following an observation, there are some critical points to follow when writing field-notes to minimize loss of data. These include: getting right to the task; not talking about the observation before it is recorded; finding a quiet place to write; setting aside adequate time to complete the notes; sequencing events in the order they occurred; and letting the events and conversation flow from the mind on to the paper. If something is forgotten, it can always be added to the notes later.

· One point the researcher must consider is that it takes nearly three times as long to record the observation as it does to do the observation. This is one reason why using a tape recorder is preferred, as it is faster for the researcher to dictate the observations into the recorder.

The process of writing field-notes

Field-notes consist of jottings of salient points that are reworked in detail later the same day. They take the form of reconstructions of interactions, short conversational excerpts or descriptions of events. The notes recorded during an interaction are kept brief so that the observer can concentrate on what is happening in order to get the feeling of the situation as well as the actual verbal exchange. Field-notes are also used to identify ideas on relationships within the data, which then provide a beginning cross-check for later analysis.

Field-notes are a written account of the things that the researcher hears, sees, experiences and thinks in the course of collecting or reflecting on data in a qualitative study (Bogdan and Biklen, 1982). Detailed, accurate and extensive field-notes are necessary for a successful qualitative study. In studies which use participant observation, all data are recorded as field-notes.

Field-notes may also be used to supplement other forms of data gathering. A tape-recorded interview does not portray the physical setting, the impressions the observer picks up or the non-verbal communication in an observed interaction. These observations should be recorded in field-notes to supplement the taped interview. During the course of the observations, the researcher may become aware of subjective biases and unsubstantiated hunches relating to the setting or the phenomena. It is important to keep track of early hunches as they may later prove to be erroneous. While some researchers advocate using field-notes to record these impressions, it may be preferable to record them in a separate diary. In this way objective and subjective records are maintained separately. Furthermore, field-notes may become public property and used by future researchers. Therefore it is less inhibiting if it is known that these early impressions will remain within the researcher's own files.

The content of field-notes

As mentioned, field-notes are descriptive accounts in which the researcher objectively records what is happening in the setting. The researcher's goal is to capture the lived experience of the participants and to describe the community of which they are a part. It is unrealistic to expect that all aspects of a setting can be described, but it is important to record as much as possible in the field-notes, guided, in part, by the project's research goals.

In field-notes it is necessary to quote what people say rather than to summarize their words. If one is observing a nurse providing care, it would be important to describe what that care entailed. For example an entry may read:

> The nurse spoke to the patient, 'How are you today, Mrs B.?'; did not wait for a reply, turned back the bedclothes and inspected the dressing.

This provides a more accurate description than saying, 'checked the patient'. It is critical not to mix evaluation of actions with a description of care. If the observer stated, 'The nurse made a superficial check', the observer has placed a value on the action by using the word 'superficial'. This leads to the observer glossing over actions rather than dissecting them and searching for the meaning of the action or the reason behind the action.

Field-notes will encompass varying areas. The notes may include portraits of subjects, which involve describing physical appearance, dress, mannerisms or style of talking. Any facet of appearance or behaviour which sets an individual apart from the group should be noted.

Another important area to record is reconstruction of dialogue. This resembles nurses' process recordings and may be between participants or between participants and the researcher. Both public conversations and private dialogue may be recorded. Non-verbal communication, such as gestures and facial expression, should also be noted. When the reconstructed dialogue is only a close approximation of what was said, square brackets or other selected identifiers should be used to indicate this in the notes. If it is questionable as to whether or not a passage is accurately recorded, this should also be indicated in the notes.

In describing a transcultural situation, the researcher may want to make detailed notes of subtle differences in behaviour. For example the mother may approach bathing a newborn in a way unfamiliar to the observer. A note of the behaviours involved may be needed to recall the details of the activity, because once the researcher becomes familiar with the setting such differences may no longer be apparent.

In a hospital setting, the relationships among the family may require an account of a particular event. If food is brought by the family, who brings it? Of what does the food consist? Are there rituals to be observed prior to eating? The event, the manner in which the event occurred, as well as behaviours specific to the act, should all be recorded.

In another example, Soares (1978), in recording the communication patterns in an intensive care unit, provided details of a communication event. She described the stimulus for the communication, the persons engaged in the communication, the level and tone of voice, and the behaviour of the participants. Rich data recorded in the field-notes is filled with pieces of evidence that enable the researcher to identify clues that begin to make analytical sense of the data that is studied.

The observer also needs to note any behaviours that may have affected the observation. Actions and conversations which may have changed the interaction must be recorded. The influence of the researcher on the setting should be minimized, but, as there will always be some impact, keeping a careful record can help in the assessment of untoward influences.

In addition to descriptive material, the observer may record sentences and paragraphs that reflect a less objective account of the incident and serve as memos. A notation, such as 'OC' (observer's comments), may be used to identify the observer's feelings, problems, hunches, impressions or prejudices, and any ethical dilemmas or conflicts (Bogdan and Taylor, 1975). The researcher may also indicate areas that need clarification or potential misunderstandings between the observer and participant.

The form of field-notes

Field-notes may either be spoken into a tape recorder for later transcription or recorded in written form. For the latter method, a small, neutral-coloured loose-leaf notebook is one of the easiest ways of recording field-notes. It is easily portable and is relatively unobtrusive in use. The notes for each subject can be filed directly into a master file. Dating pages is often of more value than numbering them in keeping track of observations. A second notebook, with pockets, can be used to store consent forms, information sheets, activity sheets and observation and interview schedules, if appropriate. It can also be used to keep track of the progress of the research.

For each separate observation session recorded in the field-notes, it is wise to record the site at which the observation took place, the date and time of the observation, who made the observation and the number of this set of notes in the total study (Figure 5.1). This information should be cross-referenced to the researcher's observation and/or interview schedule, as this acts as an aid in keeping track of the data and locating related observations or interviews.

Participant Code #

Interview date   Starting time   Ending time

Pre-interview goals for interview

Location of interview

People present

Description of environment (including personal belongings, etc.)

Non-verbal behaviour (e.g. tone of voice, posture, facial expressions, eye movement, forcefulness of speech, body movement, hand gestures)

Content of interview (e.g. use of keywords, topics, focus, exact words or phrases which stand out)

Researcher's impressions (e.g. discomfort of participant with certain topics, emotional responses to people, events or objects)

Analysis (e.g. researcher's questions, tentative hunches, trends in data, emerging patterns)

Technological problems (e.g. lost 5 minutes when tape turned)

Figure 5.1 A sample format for recording field-notes

MAPS

Drawings to show placement of furniture or people during a particular event may also be included in field-notes. Physical maps describe arrangements and layouts, physical patterns in the environment and listing of significant objects in a setting. This information may be obtained through observation and through questioning the participants about the significance of observed objects in the setting.

The use of maps in research is particularly appropriate when the movements of persons in social space are relevant to the location and movement of the same persons in physical space (Melbin, 1960). Diagrams (such as sociograms), floor plans, flow charts and aerial photographs may all be considered maps for research purposes.

For example in Toohey's study of an emergency department, she demonstrated that the physical structure of the setting allowed the nurses to set the stage in such a way that they appeared to be busy to the patients at times when activity in the emergency department was actually low. The structure also allowed the nurses to avoid sustained contact with patients who were not seen as true emergencies (Toohey and Field, 1985). It was critical to develop maps of the department early in the study in order to identify the relationship between physical and social space.

ADDITIONAL METHODS OF DATA COLLECTION

Life histories, diaries, analysis of personal collections, and study of official documents may be used alone or in conjunction with participant observation. Life histories use interviewing techniques and can be considered as a specialized form of interview. Official documents or hard data, such as census information, are used on occasion to verify data provided by participants, and may be employed as one method of triangulation.

Life history

A life history is used when a researcher wants to explore the history of an individual (micro-history) within a framework of time (macro-history). A life history enables the researcher to explore an individual's current attitudes and behaviours while giving consideration to decisions that were made at an earlier point in time and potentially in another place. Life histories may be first-person narratives structured according to a chronological sequence.

Life histories differ from biographies in that the purpose of a biography is to learn about the details of the life of an individual, usually someone who is well known in a particular society or culture. Bogdan and Taylor (1975) suggest that a life history will require 50–60 hours of interview, comprised of weekly interviews over a five-month period. In contrast, oral histories may be obtained with relatively short interview periods, for example three to four hours divided between two sessions (Safier, 1977).

Both life histories and oral histories attempt to determine the attitudes and behaviours of an individual over time. However, the purpose of the life history is to embed the life history of the individual within the context of their life experience, which potentially takes more time than obtaining a straight oral history of an individual's life. This latter tends to be more similar to a biography than a life history. It is recognized that in the literature the terms **life history**, **oral history** and **biography** may be used interchangeably (Hagermaster, 1992), but it is critical that those claiming to use a life history understand the purpose and method.

In selecting a sample for a life history, it is critical to remember that while everyone has a story to tell, that story may not be appropriate for a life history. It is critical that the participant has the time to commit to the project and is willing to talk about his/her life from the perspective of interest to the researcher. One key to a successful life history is the rapport developed between the researcher and participant. A trusting relationship will be critical to success.

Ethical concerns arise in life-history research. The first is the protection of anonymity when in-depth information is obtained from individuals. It is difficult to write a detailed report without risk of identification of individuals. Because a long-term relationship is involved, the researcher may risk becoming over-involved in the life of the participant and may become a counsellor rather than a researcher. If the study is on vulnerable individuals (such as battered women), conflict may develop between therapeutic and research needs.

A life history is potentially a valid form of data collection. As data are collected over a long period of time, questions can be rephrased and answers restated and comparisons of response made over time.

Both tape-recorded interviews and field-notes are used in a life history. Data may be gathered through the use of both direct and indirect questions. Descriptive, structural and contrast questions are all used to elicit information and are used throughout the study. Actual events in an individual's life may be used to develop a chronology. In this process, both dates and an individual's age may be used. When identified, major turning points in an individual's life may form the basis for further interview questions.

Data analysis uses coding, categorizing, and clustering of themes, as with ethnographic research (Miles and Huberman, 1994). The researcher will compare patterns of life experience across participants. Conceptual frameworks may be useful in organizing emerging data, for example career histories may be used to help explain the career patterns of nurse leaders. Care must be taken, however, that the framework is not used to control the data.

Life histories could be useful in explaining shared behavioural and belief patterns both within and across cultures. Use of life histories could demonstrate the evolution of career patterns or explain how patients learn to cope with chronic illness over time. A researcher who wants to use life history as a method of data gathering needs to recognize that the process is time-consuming and carries the risks of emotional involvement developing with the participant over time. Reconstituting one's early years may be difficult. Photographs and other family documents can be used to jar the participant's memory. This type of research requires considerable time commitment and cooperation from the participants.

When obtaining a life history, it is critical that the participant's own words be used. Tape recording is normally essential for data collection. However, if tape recording is not possible, nurses have usually had extensive experience in process recording interactions, and it is appropriate to utilize these skills at this time. One instance where process recording can be used is in the case of an individual whose testimony may put him/her at risk. This would particularly apply if the individual could be recognized from the recorded voice. Languess (1965) elaborates on the ethics of writing a life history and identifies safeguards for researcher and participant, and it is a useful reference source for those seeking more detailed information.

Life histories of new immigrants would enable the helping professions to better understand the problems of migration and culture shock. Life histories of some of the early pioneer nurses would add another dimension to the understanding of the evolution of nursing over the last century. The impact of severe or disabling illness on a person's life could be examined through life history techniques.

Diaries

Diaries may be a useful source of data and can provide an intimate descriptive comment on everyday life for an individual. A researcher may use personal diaries that have been kept by an individual on a daily basis. This is a resource that has been used by both historians and biographers to recapitulate and provide insight into an individual's life.

The use of a diary is a technique that has been used by social scientists in a variety of research endeavours. In the past few years, diaries have been reported as a primary method of data collection in some research reports (Ross, Rideout and Carson, 1994).

Diaries can be used as either a semi-structured or unstructured method of data collection. Most frequently the researcher provides some structure by asking participants to record particular information in relation to some aspect of a specific experience or event. Diaries have been used in health-related research with some success (Freer, 1980, Hickey, Akingama and Rakowski, 1991; Ross, Rideout and Carson, 1994). They have been used both as a primary source of data (Ross, Rideout and Carson, 1994) and to verify data

(O'Hare, 1991). Respondent cooperation and quality of data have been found to be very satisfactory (Verbrugge, 1980).

Quality of data in diaries should not be influenced by recall, as events are recorded close to the event being described. It does, however, require sustained respondent cooperation. Diary use has generally been reported in studies with middle-income families where the participants have a high-school education. This may have been a factor in the high level of cooperation and the quality of data. Diaries appear to be a useful way of collecting data, but, as their use is relatively new, continued monitoring of the quality of data and the co-operation of participants is essential.

Photographs

Photographs can provide researchers with visual images of a context. They can also be used to provide visual insights and knowledge about human conditions.

Photographs may stimulate a participant's recall of an event, thus leading to richer data and greater understanding of the event by the researcher. Events can be captured and later reflected upon and interpreted to explore the meaning of the event for the participant. This both enriches and develops the communication of the experience between the participant and the researcher. The advantage of using photographs in this way is that they enable the participant to tell a story in a spontaneous manner, particularly when the exploration focuses on the compassionate dimensions of human experience, such as in Highley's (1989) work on caring behaviours within the family. Hagedorn (1990) also describes the use of photography in nursing research.

Letters and personal documents

Personal letters provide rich data that are helpful in revealing relationships between people who correspond. Letters from patients to their families could also provide insights into the hospital experience. Historically, many of the published biographies of Florence Nightingale have relied heavily on both her personal and private letters as one source of data for describing her life and career (Woodham-Smith, 1983). Personal letters from many individuals may be combined and analysed to understand an event or phenomenon. The analysis of suicide notes (Lester and Reeve, 1982) is an example of this type of research.

Official documents

In health care research, the most commonly used types of official documents are vital statistics, health care statistics, hospital statistics and patient/client records. Hospitals and health care agencies keep and generate tremendous amounts of qualitative and quantitative data. Quantitative data, such as patient statistics, can be useful in showing trends in care. Statistics may also be used to support the representativeness of the participants in a qualitative study in relation to the social group being studied when this information is of use. Statistical data may also be used to check impressions. For example if the observer in an out-patient setting sees very few children, this observation can be checked against attendance statistics, thus validating the observation. The researcher might then seek for an explanation of this finding: 'Why do few children attend out-patient clinics for care?'

In qualitative research, patient records can also be used to validate information provided by patients and nurses about treatment or medical intervention on a given unit. Charts may also be the primary unit of analysis for qualitative researchers interested in examining certain trends. One example would be analysis of Kardex$^{©}$ to explore the 'labels' nurses give to patients.

Other official documents may be formal admission or discharge interviews. Cohen (1981) studied students who left nursing without completing an educational programme. She compared entry grades and school marks with five years of exit interviews and found under-achievement was related to emotional problems and an inability to accept the nurse's role and not to a lack of intellectual potential.

PRINCIPLES

- Participants should select both the time and the place of the interview.
- Establish rapport before the interview begins.
- When using unstructured interactive interviews, let the participants tell their stories; the researcher's role is to listen.
- Allow the participant to determine where the story begins and the sequence of the story.
- The researcher is not a counsellor; listen attentively, but do not intervene.
- Semi-structured interviews are used when the researcher knows the questions but cannot determine the answers.
- Short-answer, open-ended written questionnaires can be used to collect data when some dimensions of the phenomena are known.
- Observation adds breadth to the interview and provides answers to contextual questions that cannot be answered by interview alone.
- A research setting should be separate from one's work setting.
- Behaviour may be changed in the presence of an observer, but adequate time may reduce this threat.
- Field-notes are critical in qualitative research and should be completed as soon as possible after the event occurred.
- Other data collection techniques, such as maps, life histories, photographs, letters, diaries and personal and official documents may enrich the data.

REFERENCES

Bogdan, R. and Biklen, S.K. (1982) *Qualitative Research for Education: An Introduction to Theory and Methods*, Allyn and Bacon, Toronto.

Bogdan, R.C. and Taylor, S.J. (1975) *Introduction to Qualitative Research Methods: A Phenomenological Approach to the Social Sciences*, John Wiley and Sons, New York.

Campbell, I.E., Larrivee, L., Field, P.A. *et al.* (1994) Learning to nurse in the clinical setting. *Advanced Journal of Nursing*, **20**, pp. 1125–31.

Cohen, H.A. (1981) *The Nurse's Quest for a Professional Identity*, Addison-Wesley, Menlo Park, CA.

Davis, D.L. (1986/92) The meaning of menopause in a Newfoundland fishing village, in *Qualitative Health Research*, (ed. J.M. Morse), Sage, Newbury Park, CA, pp. 145–69.

Doan, H. and Morse, J.M. (1985) The last taboo: roadblocks for researching menarche. *Health Care for Women International*, **6**(5–6), 277–83.

Freer, C.B. (1980) Self care: a health care study. *Medical Care*, **18**, 835–61.

Golander, H. (1987/92) Under the guise of passivity, in *Qualitative Health Research*, (ed. J.M. Morse), Sage, Newbury Park, CA, pp. 192–201.

Gold, R.L. (1958) Roles in sociological observation. *Social Forces*, **36**, 217–23.

Hagedorn, M. (1990) Using photography with families of chronically ill children, in *The Caring Imperative in Education*, (eds M. Leininger and J. Watson), The National League for Nursing, New York, pp. 227–34.

Hagermaster, J.N. (1992) Life history: a qualitative method of research. *Journal of Advanced Nursing*, **17**, 1122–8.

Hickey, T., Akingama, H. and Rakowski, W. (1991) The illness characteristics and health care decisions of older people. *Journal of Applied Gerontology*, **10**, 169–83.

Highley, B. (1989) The camera in nursing research and practice, in *Toward a Science of Family Nursing*, (eds C. Gilliss, B. Highly, B. Roberts and I.M. Martinson), Addison-Wesley, Menlo Park, CA, pp. xxi – xxvii.

Languess, L.C. (1965) *The Life History in Anthropological Science*, Holt, Rinehart and Winston, New York.

Leininger, M. (1985) Nature, rationale and importance of qualitative research methods in nursing, in *Qualitative Research Methods in Nursing*, (ed. M. Leininger), Grune and Stratton, London, pp. 1–26.

Lester, D. and Reeve, C. (1982) The suicide notes of young and old people. *Psychological Reports*, **50**, 334.

Melbin, M. (1960) Mapping uses and methods, in *Human Organization Research: Field Relations and Techniques* (eds R.N. Adams and J.J. Preiss), Dorsey Press, Homewood, IL, pp. 255–66.

Miles, N.B. and Huberman, A.B. (1994) *Qualitative Data Analysis*, 2nd edn, Sage, Thousand Oaks, CA.

Morse, J.M. (1984) Cultural context of infant feeding in Fiji. *Ecology of Food and Nutrition*, **14**, 287–96.

Morse, J.M. and Bottorff, J.L. (1988/92) The emotional experience of breast expression, in *Qualitative Health Research*, (ed. J.M. Morse), Sage, Menlo Park, CA, pp. 319–32.

Morse, J.M. and Bottorff, J.L. (1989a) Intending to breastfeed and work. *Journal of Obstetrical, Gynecological and Neonetal Nursing*, **18**(6), 493–500.

Morse, J.M. and Bottorff, J.L. (1989b) Managing breastfeeding: the problem of leaking. *Journal of Nurse Midwifery*, **34**(1), 15–20.

Norris, J. (1991) Mothers' involvement in their adolescent daughters' abortions, in *The Illness Experience*, (eds J.M. Morse and J.L. Johnson), Sage, Newbury Park, CA, pp. 201–36.

Nystrom, A.E.M. and Segesten, K.M. (1994) On source of powerlessness in nursing home life. *Journal of Advanced Nursing*, **19**, 124–33.

O'Hare, T. (1991) Measuring alcohol consumption: a comparison of the retrospective diary and the quantity – frequency methods in a college drinking survey. *Journal of Studies on Alcohol*, **52**, 500–2.

Paterson, B.L. (1994) A framework to identify reactivity in qualitative research. *Western Journal of Nursing Research*, **16**, 301–16.

Pearsall, M. (1965) Participant observation as a role and method in behavioral research. *Nursing Research*, **14**(1), 37–42.

Rosenhan, D.L. (1973/92) On being sane in insane places, in *Qualitative Health Research*, (ed. J.M. Morse), Sage, Menlo Park, CA, pp. 202–24.

Ross, M.M., Rideout, E.M. and Carson, M.M. (1994) The use of the diary as a data collection technique. *Western Journal of Nursing Research*, **16**, 414–25.

Safier, G. (1977) *Contemporary American Leaders in Nursing: An Oral History*, McGraw-Hill, New York.

Soares, C.A. (1978) Low verbal use and status maintenance amongst intensive care nurses, in *The Nursing Profession: Views Through the Mist*, (ed. N.L. Chaska), McGraw-Hill, New York, pp. 198–204.

Toohey, S. and Field, P.A. (1985) Parents' descriptions of care. *Nursing Mirror*, **161**(19), 38–40.

Verbrugge, L. (1980) Health diaries. *Medical Care*, **18**, 73–95.

Wax, R. (1971) *Doing Fieldwork: Warnings and Advice*, University of Chicago Press, Chicago.

Weinholz, D. (1991) The study of physicians during attending rounds: a study of team learning among medical students. *Qualitative Health Research*, **1**, 152–77.

Woodham-Smith, C. (1983) *Florence Nightingale 1820–1910*, Atheneum, New York.

FURTHER READING

Adler, P.A. and Adler, P. (1987) *Membership Roles in Field Research*, Sage, Newbury Park, CA.

Basch, C.E. (1987) Focus group interview: an under-utilized research technique for improving theory and practice in health education. *Health Education Quarterly*, **14**, 411–48.

Bauer, P.F. (1984) Personal reflections on participant observation as a methodology in the social sciences. *Pastoral Psychology*, **32**, 140–5.

Denzin, N.K. (1989) *Interpretive Biography*, Sage, Newbury Park, CA.

Fine, G.A. and Sandstrom, K.L. (1988) *Knowing Children: Participant Observation with Minors*, Sage, Newbury Park, CA.

Harel, I. (1991) The silent observer and holistic note-taker: using video for documenting a research project, in *Constructionism*, (eds I. Harel and S. Papert), Ablex, Norwood, pp. 449–64.

Ives, E.D. (1974) *The Tape-Recorded Interview: A Manual for Field Workers and Oral History*, The University of Tennessee Press, Knoxville.

Krueger, R.A. (1994) *Focus Groups: A Practical Guide for Applied Research*, 2nd edn, Sage, Thousand Oaks, CA.

McCracken, G. (1988) *The Long Interview*, Sage, Newbury Park, CA.

Nyamathi, A. and Shuler, P. (1990) Focus group interview: a research technique for informed nursing practice. *Journal of Advanced Nursing*, **15**, 1281–8.

Richardson, A. (1994) The health diary: an examination of its use as a data collection method. *Journal of Advanced Nursing*, **19**, 782–91.

Rogers, A.E., Caruso, C.C. and Aldrich, M.S. (1993) Reliability of sleep diaries for assessment of sleep/wake patterns. *Nursing Research*, **42**, 368–72.

Schein, E.H. (1987) *The Clinical Perspective in Fieldwork*, Sage, Newbury Park, CA.

Schwartzman, H.B. (1993) *Ethnography in Organizations*, Sage, Newbury Park, CA.

Stafford, M.R. and Stafford, T.F. (1993) Participant observation and the pursuit of truth: methodological and ethical considerations. *Journal of the Market Research Society*, **35**, 63–76.

Thomas, J. (1993) *Doing Critical Ethnography*, Sage, Newbury Park, CA.

Principles of data analysis | 6

Two components of the research process complement each other to ensure that the finished product is excellent qualitative research. The first is the collection of adequate and appropriate data, and the second is creativity in data analysis. In this chapter, the process of creative data analysis will be addressed. First, the cognitive process of doing qualitative data analysis will be presented. Next, data preparation and data management techniques that facilitate analysis will be described, and last, procedures to verify the analysis process (i.e. an audit trail) and procedures of verifying the emerging theory will be presented.

THE PROCESS OF ANALYSIS

For the investigator, qualitative inquiry is an active process (Morse, 1994). Theory does not 'emerge from data' without immersion and complete familiarity with the data, and without active intellectual work. If the researcher is lucky enough to experience insight, then it is because adequate work has been done to prepare the data in a form that enhances the recognition of patterns, and the researcher has worked to 'prepare the mind'. On the part of the researcher, creative and solid data analysis requires astute questioning, a relentless search for answers, active observation and accurate recall. It is a process of fitting data together, of making the invisible obvious, of linking and attributing consequences to antecedents. It is a process of conjecture and verification, of correction and modification, of suggestion and defence.

Four cognitive processes appear integral to all qualitative methods: **comprehending, synthesizing (decontexualizing), theorizing**, and **recontextualizing**. These processes occur more or less sequentially, for the researcher must reach a reasonable level of comprehension before being able to synthesize (i.e. to make generalized statements about the participants), and until the researcher is able to synthesize, theorizing is not possible. Recontextualization cannot occur until the concepts or models in the investigation are fully developed.

Experienced researchers are able to set up the database so that the transitions from one process to another are achieved with ease. In addition, some looping back and forward is inevitable as, for instance some gaps in comprehension may be discovered if some areas of the database seem uneven and more data are needed in order to achieve saturation. In such cases, data collection may be resumed. As the inquiry progresses, it is possible to work on several categories or research problems simultaneously.

Comprehending

While the researcher is collecting data, it is crucial to keep the literature 'in abeyance' and at all times separate from the data to prevent 'contamination'. Participants' categories may not be identical to well-established concepts described in the literature, so the labels must be selected cautiously. If the researcher chooses to use an identical label to describe the behaviour, the description of the term must be complete and must include a comparative analysis of how it resembles or is dissimilar from the ways other authors use the term. The theory obtained from the literature is used as a template for comparison, so the researcher may recognize what is new and exciting in the data, and recognize instantly something that is known.

As soon as data collection begins, the researcher begins preparing data for analysis. Interviews are transcribed, checked, corrected and coded. Gradually, as the researcher makes sense of the setting and learns what is going on, data analysis as the process of **making sense of the data** begins. The stage of **comprehension** is reached when the researcher has enough data to be able to write a complete, detailed, coherent and rich description.

The processes of data **analysis** facilitates comprehension. Coding as a central process not only helps the researcher to sort the data, it helps the researcher to uncover underlying meanings in the text and metaphorical references, and it brings both the central and peripheral referents to the researcher's attention. Intraparticipant microanalysis, or line-by-line (and sometimes word-by-word) analysis of an interview transcript from one partici-pant, is the primary mechanism by which this is achieved. When coding line by line, Pierce's (1931, cited in Atkinson, 1990, p. 84) signs (i.e. the **icon**, the **index** and the **symbol**) are useful. These distinguish the relations between the sign and what it signifies, as follows: the **icon** is dependent on the relationship of the sign and what is signified, with an iconic relationship based upon qualities between the two; the **index** is a sign that points to something else, indicating causality; and a **symbol** represents an arbitrary relationship between the sign and its representation. Thus, established theory is used as a 'backdrop' to sensitize and illuminate the data or to enlighten the researcher.

When comprehension is reached, the researcher is able to identify stories that are a part of the topic, identify patterns of experience and predict their outcome. When little new is learned, when the interviewer has heard 'everything' and is bored, then saturation is reached and **comprehending** is completed.

Synthesizing

Synthesizing is the 'sifting' part of the analysis, and it begins when the investigator is 'getting a feel' for the setting. This is the stage when the investigator can describe the norms eloquently (such as 'these folk do this and that') and have some notion about the range and variation of behaviours. Researchers have reached this level in the data collection when they can describe 'aggregate' stories of 'how these people do ...'. Tripp-Reimer and Cohen (1991) describe synthesizing as rather like 'taking an average'. Indications that the stage of synthesis has been reached are the ability to provide, with confidence, composite descriptions of how people act or have the ability to relate or respond when suffering, without referring to notes and with the ability to provide specific stories as examples to illustrate the generalization.

When synthesizing, certain points of juncture, or critical factors, reveal themselves as significant and permit the person to explain variation in the data. It is important that these factors **earn** their way into the data set and are not placed there by some inappropriate response, such as by virtue of demographics. For this reason, critical factors are usually non-traditional variables and are difficult to identify. They may be an event, an attitude, a short event or an event that takes place over a long period of time.

In qualitative inquiry, whether the researcher uses a computer program for qualitative analysis or 'cuts and pastes' by hand, the process of analysis facilitates synthesizing. Data analysis usually assumes two mechanical forms: (1) interparticipant analysis, or the comparison of transcripts from several participants; and (2) the analysis of categories, sorted by commonalties, consisting of segments of transcripts or notes compiled from transcripts of several participants. Each form of analysis facilitates cognitive processes that enable the researcher to synthesize and, as the research process continues, to interpret, to link (both with data and with other concepts), to see relationships, to conjecture and to verify findings.

Theorizing

Theory is an essential **tool** (Morse, 1992) critical to all methods of inquiry, and the fact that theorizing is a critical component of qualitative inquiry is rarely mentioned. Without theory, qualitative results would be without structure, without application, and would be disconnected from the greater body of knowledge.

Theorizing may be considered the sorting phase of the analysis. Briefly, it is the systematic selection and 'fitting' of alternative models to the data. Theorizing is the process of constructing alternative explanations and holding these against the data until the best fit that explains the data most simply is obtained.

Unfortunately, the theoretical organization of data is not passively acquired in moments of blinding insight. It is earned through an active, continuous and rigorous process of viewing data as a puzzle. Theorizing is the constant development and manipulation of data into malleable theoretical schemes until the 'best' theoretical scheme is developed. It is a process of speculation and conjecture, of falsification and verification, of selecting, revising and discarding. If one ever finishes, the final 'solution' is the theory that provides the best comprehensive, coherent and simple model for linking diverse and unrelated facts in a useful, pragmatic way. It is a way of revealing the obvious, the implicit, the unrecognized, the unknown. It is a way of discovering the insignificance of the significant and the significance of the insignificant.

An example of a study in which theorizing was used is Morse's (1991/92) 'Negotiating commitment and involvement in the patient–nurse relationship'. A model depicting the differences in time spent with the patient, style of interaction, patients' needs and type of trust which vary for four types of nurse–patient relationships are evident in the type of commitment of the nurse to the patient.

The process of data collection and analysis cannot be rushed (Glaser, 1979). Until the researcher reaches maturity through comprehension and synthesizing, the researcher must remain open to alternative modes of sorting — to alternate theories — and be wary of being wed to one explanation too early because this leads to 'premature closure'. If premature closure occurs, the resulting theory may have gaps, be thin, be weak and may even be wrong.

The first step in theorizing is to ask questions of the data that will create links to established theory. Several strategies may be used; the first is to identify the beliefs and values in the data. This strategy may, for example, establish **emic–etic** or **macro–micro** linkages from the data to theory, from the participant's perspective to a described world view. If correct, such linkages greatly speed the analysis. The second method is to use **lateral thinking** by examining similar concepts in other settings or seeking other complementary data sources in other contexts. The third method is the systematic and inductive incremental development of substantive or formal theory from the data. The last method may use conjecture and falsification, by systematically hypothesizing causal links or the sequencing of characteristics that may be attributed to certain behaviours or experiences. Key to this process is the technique of theoretical sampling, whereby characteristics suspected to contribute to an experience are identified in certain participants, who are then located and interviewed to verify or to refute the hunch.

Recontextualizing

In the process of recontextualizing, the real power of qualitative research is recognised. Recontextualization is the development of the emerging theory so that the theory is applicable to other settings and to other populations. In qualitative research, the theory is the most important product: it is, therefore, the **theory** that is generalized and recontexualized into different settings. In addition, it is the theoretical elegance that makes qualitative inquiry generalizable and gives it power in the process of recontextualisation.

It is in the process of recontextualization that the published work of other researchers and established theory plays a critical role. Established theory may provide the context in which a researcher's model links the new findings to the literature. Established theory recontextualizes the new findings by providing a context in which to fit the new findings, and thus the discipline advances. Finally, the literature provides a mechanism that assists to demonstrate the usefulness and implications of the findings. The goal is to be able to place the results in the context of established knowledge and to clearly identify those results that support the literature or clearly claim new contributions.

DATA PREPARATION

There are many different styles of qualitative research and many different approaches to handling the data, but similar processes are involved to ensure that analysis takes place in an orderly fashion. Data, in qualitative analysis, are usually in the form of textual narrative (derived from transcribed interviews); written descriptions of observations (as field-notes); and reflections, ideas and conjectures recorded in the researcher's diary. These records are usually voluminous. An audiotaped, 45-minute interview, for instance may result in 25 pages of text to be checked, coded, sorted and stored in a form that may be easily retrieved and analysed.

Transcribing interviews

The first major task in analysing interview data is to become extremely familiar with the data. As soon as possible after the completion of a tape-recorded interview, the tape should be replayed with the researcher listening carefully to the content as well as to the questions asked and to the participant's response. As noted in Chapter 5, field-notes are written at this time to describe the interview context. Duplicate the tape, so that if the tape is damaged — or accidentally erased — in the process of transcribing, a backup will be available.

Next, the tape is transcribed directly into the computer, in the form that will make it readily available for analysis. It is crucial that the tape be transcribed exactly (word for word) from the interview and not paraphrased. The only exceptions are any identifying information such as names of significant others that the participant may have used. Ask the typist to indicate such identifying information was used by inserting a line, and the relationship of the person (for example: _____ [mother]). Pauses should be indicated using dashes, while an ellipse indicates gaps or prolonged pauses. All expression, including exclamations, laughter, crying and expletives, are included in the text and separated from the verbal text with square brackets. Type the interviews single-spaced with a blank line between each speaker. A generous margin on both sides of the page permits the left margin to be used for coding and the researcher's own critique of the interview style, and the right margin to be used for comments regarding the content. Transcribing is a time-consuming task, yet one that enables the interviewer to intimately know his/her data.

The transcription is then checked against the tape for accuracy. Changes in voice or tone, significant pauses and inflections that may indicate that the topic is highly important or emotionally charged become lost in transcribing. Place researcher-comments directly into the transcript, using a **Bold** font to separate it from the actual interview text. Ensure all pages are numbered sequentially and that each page is coded with the interview number and participant's number. Finally, and most importantly, print and back up the computer file!

Managing such a database is an immense task which may be fraught with frustration when attempting to make sense of the data while, at the same time, endeavouring to locate a description to illustrate a particular concept or event. The purpose of data analysis is, therefore, twofold. The first purpose is to code the data so that the categories may be recognized and analysed, and behaviours noted. The second is to develop a data filing system that will provide a flexible storage system with procedures for retrieving the data. It is our experience that some new researchers have been dissatisfied with 'set' instructions for analysing data and have developed their own. General principles will be described, rather than presenting rigid procedures.

METHODS OF CODING

By the time the researcher has conducted the interview, listened to the tape and checked the transcript, she/he will be able to recognize the persistent words, phrases or themes within the data. The task of coding becomes one of identifying these words, passages or paragraphs for later retrieval and resorting.

Several ways to manage a coding system existed before the advent of the microcomputer. The most common was to label the major theme within each paragraph by writing the category in the margin, and then to sort the data by cutting each labelled paragraph and pasting or copying the relevant passage on to larger sheets of paper or on to index cards for manual sorting. Highlighting the relevant phrases assisted in sorting these portions of text into common piles in the next phase of the analysis.

Categories are initially kept as broad as possible without overlapping. Therefore few categories are chosen in the initial stages of the analysis. Then, as more data accumulates, the major categories may be sorted into smaller categories. This **rule of parsimony** enables the data to remain manageable and permits subcategories to be derived from the larger domain. Experience has shown that it is difficult during the initial data coding stage to work with more than ten major codes and still keep the codes distinct.

How are codes derived from the data? As each unit of data is examined, certain words or phrases demand the researcher's attention. For instance in a study exploring how new mothers who planned to returned to work were able to maintain breast-feeding, Morse and Bottorff (1989) asked mothers how long they planned to nurse their infants. Rather than giving a direct answer, mothers responded almost evasively, weighing the experience of others and their own past experience, knowing that such decisions were really 'as long as the infant was interested'.

> Mother: Well, as long as she [baby] is interested. You know, however long that is. That's hard to say. Kind of, you know, whatever the baby wants. I talked to a couple of the mothers up here, and one said once they started giving him the bottle, they found it easier because he had to suck pretty hard to get the letdown reflex. I've always felt that mine's fairly strong. But with my other daughter ...

Initially, quotations such as the one above would be placed in a category labelled 'Timing of breast-feeding'. However, when the responses of the rest of the sample were added, and this category became filled, the indecisive response of the mother above appeared typical. None of the mothers could really tell us how long they intended to breast-feed and work. They used phrases such as 'see if I can train him', 'thinking, maybe, tentative, September'; 'as long as I can', 'I'll see what happens when I'm at work', 'I would like to go on as long as possible', 'I'll see how it works out', 'Oh, I don't know — however, long he is interested, I suppose' and 'I'm playing it by ear'. From the above, it was clear that mothers, even though they had learned from others and from past experience, 'let' the infant select the time of weaning. The comment 'playing it by ear' from one participant appeared to capture the essence of this experience, with the careful weighing of the pros and cons, the systematic anticipation of problems and solutions should the problem actually occur. Thus, the theme was labelled, 'playing it by ear', and the characteristics that were indicative of the process were then identified.

DATA MANAGEMENT TECHNIQUES

Planning the technical aspect of data analysis and data management requires some reflection and planning. Over the last five years a number of programs have been developed for the computer-assisted analysis of textual data, and new versions of these programs are being released on a regular basis. Therefore, rather than reviewing these programs and comparing their capabilities, considerations for choosing a method for analysis will be discussed.

(For a review of computer programs, see Weitzman and Miles, 1995.) Major considerations for selecting a method include: (1) what you want to do; (2) the personal work style of the investigator; (3) how much data you will have to manage, and what form it will be in; (4) the specifics required of a program; and (5) the type of computer available for the project.

The first consideration, **what you want to do**, is inextricably linked with the method. If, for example, you wish to analyse by category, it will be necessary to select a program that permits you to insert and label a piece of text, and later copy that text from the data file to a category file that may later be labelled and named. If the investigator is using a semi-structured interview schedule, it will be necessary to categorize by item number and then by at least one level of subcategory. If the investigator is using phenomenology, then the software must have the capability of sorting by theme, as well as by each participant. With ethnographic analysis, it must be possible to categorize multiple data types in the data file by category. Finally, for grounded theory, it must be possible to include theoretical memos and diagrams illustrating linkages of data, tagged with the relevant pieces of data. The greater the amount of data, the larger the capacity of the computer. Although most microcomputers are able to manage large data sets, two programs are available for the mainframe.

Computer software

If the researcher is planning to use a computer to facilitate analysis, it is important to consider that computer programs only ease the process of **data sorting**. Computer programs facilitate the coding action: most programs minimally enable the placing of a code into the text, linked to a particular piece of data. Again, the computer does not 'code' the data — **the investigator must locate the data, recognize the significance of the data and insert the code**. The computer only merges data with the same codes into the same file. Data analysis does not occur with the pushing of a button — it takes investigator time, effort and expertise to code well.

Which program to use? Numerous programs are now available, and new versions are constantly being developed. Many texts compare the features of these programs (see Weitzman and Miles (1995) for an overview of software for textual analysis). Perhaps the most important consideration is the researcher's comfort level, first with using the computer and, secondly, the ease of using the chosen program. The program must not be so complex as to distract or overwhelm the researcher, so that rather than concentrating on the actual coding *per se*, the researcher is preoccupied with the mechanics of using the program. For medium size data sets, coding can be quite comfortably performed with a word processing program, such as Microsoft Word© (Morse, 1991). However, in order to understand the process of coding, it is recommended that the student first sort a small data set by hand.

Manual methods

The simplest method for data analysis is the use of highlighting pens which leave the typed page intact. This method, however, cannot be linked with extensive data sets. It is not possible to adequately code all the pages and to retrieve the required passages, which quickly become voluminous when multiple interviews are involved. Analysis of categories within the major constructs is extremely difficult, perhaps even impossible, with this technique. Hence, this method is not recommended for larger studies and may be problematic even when small amounts of data are involved.

The second method has been used by anthropological fieldworkers for generations. Concepts or quotes are copied on to cards and these are filed under the appropriate category. McBee cards (cards with holes punched along the top) allow easy retrieval and permit the cards to be filed under more than one category if needed. The holes pertaining to the data categories, recorded on the cards, are left intact, and those categories that are not used punched out. Retrieval is made with a metal skewer, and all cards containing the selected category may be lifted from the data set.

Goffman was rumoured to use a similar card system. It is said that he transcribed field-notes on to cards and sorted these cards by placing them in large brown envelopes. These envelopes were labelled one per category and pinned all over his office walls. Apparently, when an envelope came heavy enough to fall off the wall, there was enough data to sort into subcategories.

A third method, and the one most frequently used by the present writers, is to colour code each page of the interview in the left margin. Use one coloured stripe for each participant, and another for the interview (1, 2, 3, etc.). Then, when analysing the data, cut the significant passages from the interview, tape each piece on to a full-size sheet of paper and file it in the appropriate folder for that category. The colour coding is a fast method of identifying all data, allowing pieces coded for analysis to be traced to the original source. Cutting the transcript enables the data to be quickly sorted without the necessity of rewriting the appropriate passage on to another card. However, as one segment may fit into two or more categories, the need for several copies of data is obvious. As the file folders fill, the contents are again sorted into smaller categories.

TYPES OF ANALYSIS

In recent years the types of analyses have proliferated. Phenomenologists write of **thematic analysis** (analysing for themes), linguists of **semantic analysis** (analysing the language), and others of **content analysis**, analysing for categories, constructs, domains and so forth. Lofland (1971) makes a useful distinction between **static** and **phase analysis**. A static analysis will depict an event as it occurs. Phase analysis is used in the development of a phenomenon over a period of time. It is important for the researcher to use both forms of analysis and to identify two processes when reporting the research. Furthermore, it is necessary to link static events with one another and to demonstrate relations between such events if they exist.

Fox (1982, pp. 391–409) and Babbie (1979, p. 279) write of latent and manifest content analysis. Latent content analysis is the type most commonly used in qualitative analysis. Passages or paragraphs are reviewed in the context of the entire interview in order to identify and code the thrust or intent of the section and the significant meanings within passages. This permits the overt intent of the participant to be coded, in addition to the analysis of the underlying meanings in the communication. The method has high validity but may be less reliable due to the possible subjective nature of the coding system.

When using manifest content analysis the researcher surveys the scripts for words, phrases, descriptors and terms central to the research. These are tabulated and may be analysed using descriptive statistics. Numeric objectivity of the analysis increases the reliability of the procedure but loses validity as the technique denies the richness of the research context.

Frequently researchers use both methods in a complementary fashion. They may start with thick description and latent content analysis as categories are established and described then move on to tabulation and descriptive statistics to enumerate the number of times specific concepts are discussed or behaviours observed. Care must be taken when this technique is employed as factors such as time, verbal expressiveness or repetitions may influence the number of instances of a phenomenon being observed, and in qualitative research these variables are not constant for all participants.

CLASSIFICATION SYSTEMS

In the initial phase of the analysis the researcher attempts to identify the characteristics of observed phenomena. In making notations, the researcher should note (i) the kinds of things that are going on in the context being studied, (ii) the forms a phenomenon takes and (iii) any variations within a phenomenon.

The purpose of this analysis is to delineate the form, kinds and types of social phenomena and to document their existence. This is the naming process that results in the development of classification systems. One example of the use of a taxonomy is the Linnean taxonomy used to classify living organisms. Each category of life-form has a list of characteristics that allows scientists to place all living objects within the classification system. A taxonomy does not, however, account for processes. A taxonomy or classification system, whose function is to name objects, only creates an orderly framework for analysing the data. Within a given setting acts (one-shot events), activities (ongoing events), verbal productions that direct actions (meanings), participation of the actors, interrelationships among actions and the setting of the study may all be means of setting up a classification system.

In the anthropological tradition, the history, social structure, recurring events, economy, authority, beliefs and values of a community may constitute the initial list of universal categories used to organize data. On the other hand, categories may arise easily from the data. For example in a study of patient satisfaction with nursing care, when the participant says: 'Oh, the nurses were great but the interns — they were another matter', one already has as categories 'nurses' and 'interns'. The behaviours 'were great' and the alternative 'were another matter' indicate two areas which the researcher needs to explore further in order to understand the meaning of these phrases for the participant. From the start, the researcher will be able to record labels for categories provided by participants. If a category of 'doctors' emerges, 'interns' will become a segregate or subset of that category

Matrix formation

In examining the universals it may be useful to develop matrices to look at relationships between categories (Miles and Huberman, 1994). Development of a matrix may help to uncover the relationships between parents and the sick child, the role the nurse and physician play in this relationship (authority, decision making) and the meanings conveyed by covert rules. It may be noted that the categories developed can be related to established theoretical concepts such as kinship, group ritual and authority, but use labels that match the data as closely as possible. To note such relationships may be valuable in formulating tentative propositions and in interpreting the data. Spradley (1980, pp. 82–3) provides an excellent example of questions developed to describe a phenomenon. This example graphs all possible relationships along the dimensions of space, object, act, activity, event, time, actor, goal and feeling so that a comprehensive picture of all possible relationships is obtained.

Formulating tentative propositions

As the fieldworker collects more data, relationships among behaviours, participants, activities and so forth will begin to emerge. The researcher will develop hunches about relationships within the data and will formulate tentative propositions about these relationships. In some studies one will see the term 'proposition' used, while in others, 'research hypotheses' will be generated. A proposition is a subject to be discussed or a statement to be upheld; it is something to be assumed for the purpose of argument. A hypothesis is defined as a proposition or principle which is supposed or taken for granted in order to draw a conclusion: it is a theoretical relationship between variables imagined or assumed for the purpose of argument. The choice of term would seem to be more a matter of training than of real difference.

Propositions are stated in such a way that they indicate potential relationships within the data. They may be stated as causal propositions. For example a study on clients who attended a nurse-run clinic where the goal was health promotion yielded the following propositions (Field, 1984):

- clients who perceive themselves as having inner control over their daily activities will expect guidance and support from the nurse in response to their initiation of an interaction; and
- clients who lack inner control over their daily activities will expect the nurse to act as an authoritarian figure who exerts control.

These propositions are then used to guide further data gathering. The researcher looks for evidence that will either support or invalidate the proposition or hypothesis. Tentative propositions may be supported, may have to be amended or may need to be discarded over the course of a study. Hypotheses are a necessary part of the research process when qualitative data is to be converted to quantifiable data for analysis or if new theoretical ideas are to be generated.

ATYPICAL CASES

The researcher must distinguish between representative cases and anecdotal cases. Representative cases appear with regularity and encompass the range of behaviours described within a category. The anecdotal case appears infrequently and depicts a small range of events which are atypical of the larger group.

In the case previously cited (Field, 1984), the clients attending the nurse-run clinic who perceived that they had inner control were representative of the modal group of clients attending the clinic. The clients who lacked inner control represented the anecdotal case, their overall behaviour and characteristics were similar to that of the total population, but in this one dimension they were atypical of the larger group.

Negative cases are those episodes that clearly refute an emergent theory or proposition. Negative cases are important as they help to clarify additional causal properties which influence the phenomena under study (Denzin, 1978).

Thematic analysis

Briefly, thematic analysis involves the search for and identification of common threads that extend throughout an entire interview or set of interviews. Themes are usually quite abstract and therefore difficult to identify. Often the theme does not immediately 'jump out' of the interview, but may be more apparent if the researcher steps back and considers, 'What are these folks trying to tell me?' The theme may be beneath the surface of the interviews but, once identified, appears obvious. Frequently, these themes are concepts **indicated** by the data, rather than concrete entities directly described by the participants. For example mothers' descriptions of how they felt while their child was hospitalized may contain many stories of wanting to assist the sick child, but also descriptions of feeling that the care was under the control of the staff; of wanting to be at home with the other well children, but feeling that their responsibility was with the sick child; and of fatigue and exhaustion arising from 'doing nothing' at the hospital all day; of working intensely into the night when their husbands arrive to relieve them at the hospital and they can finally go home to their other children. The themes identified may relate to power-lessness and lack of control, protection of the sick child, conflicting roles, overload and stress. Note that in their interviews the mothers did not use the actual words of the identified theme, but, rather, throughout the interviews reiterated stories on these topics.

How does a researcher 'code' for a theme? The first task is to read and reread the interviews in their entirety. Step back and reflect on the interviews as a whole. Write memos that are general in nature, summarizing the entire inter-view, keeping in mind that more than one theme may exist in a set of interviews. Once identified, the themes appear to be significant concepts that link substan-tial portions of the interviews together.

Content analysis

Content analysis is analysis by topic, and each interview is segmented by these topics into categories. An interview segment that is separated from the inter-view may consist of a few lines or maybe more than a paragraph. Codes identify the content in the interview and category labels are descriptive names for each group of data.

When conducting content analysis, the researcher reads the entire interview and identifies several important topics in the interview. These topics then become the primary categories, or category labels. Note that the categories are initially broad, so that a large amount of data may be sorted into a few groups, usually between 10 and 15 categories per study. The reason that these categories are kept to a minimum is that if the categories are too 'specialized', very small amounts of data will fit into each category. A large number of categories will be necessary to begin the analysis, and the researcher will quickly find that many of the categories contain only one or two pieces of data and that eventually categories will have to be combined. With too many categories, saturation is achieved slowly. But the greatest problem is that the investigator cannot recall large numbers of categories and cannot sort the data effectively or efficiently.

Once the categories have ample data, the research may select to categorize these data into two or more subcategories. Thus, a tree diagram develops with 'types of' the main category. When each category is reasonably full and saturation is reached (i.e. no new data are emerging), then the researcher may write descriptive paragraphs about the categories and look for relationships between the categories. The relationships may be concurrence, antecedents or consequences of an initial category.

Question analysis

Recall that semi-structured interviews are interviews in which the participants have been asked the same questions throughout the course of the study. Thus, the analysis of this is similar to content analysis but the initial sort of the interviews is by item number. For instance all of the Question 1s are sorted into one category. From this initial sort, the investigator then reads all these responses and may conduct a content analysis of these data. If desired and if the sample size is adequate, then responses may be numerally coded and non-parametric statistics conducted to look for relationships between items or variables.

ISSUES IN QUALITATIVE RESEARCH

In any type of research, the researcher must address the issues of objectivity and subjectivity, reliability and validity. The final sections of this chapter will address these issues as they apply to qualitative methodologies.

Subjectivity

Qualitative research has been extensively criticized for the subjective nature of the methods. This subjectivity may be derived from, firstly, the researcher as an instrument, and, secondly, from the quality of the evidence or the subjective nature of the research topic.

The researcher as an instrument

In qualitative research, the amount and quality of the data and the depth of the analysis are dependent upon the ability of the researcher. For example the information elicited from an interview depends upon the ability of the interviewer to establish rapport and gain the trust of the informants or upon the researcher's interview techniques. In participant observation, the amount of information also depends upon observational skills and the amount of trust established. If trust is not present, then the setting will change when the researcher is present and participants will conceal facts from the researcher.

Finally, the depth of the data analysis will depend upon the researcher's sensitivity, perceptivity, informed value judgments, insight and knowledge.

The quality of the evidence

Qualitative researchers study people's perceptions and reports or accounts of situations and events. As such, these reports may be 'unreliable', 'biased' and contradict other reports. This is known as the 'Rashomon Effect' (Heider, 1983, p. 10) and the basis of the problems in the law courts when six witnesses may each report a different 'version of reality'. However, in qualitative research such different and discrepant perspectives are considered a part of the context, a part of the problem. For example a patient's perspective and report of a visit to the doctor may be quite different from the doctor's account of the visit, and both of these reports may differ from an objective observer's report. However, the purpose of qualitative research is not to determine objectively what actually happened (as in the court of law), but, rather, to objectively report the perceptions of each of the participants in the setting.

PROCEDURES OF VERIFICATION

Procedures of theoretical verification include verification of the emerging theory with study participants and/or with the research findings of others. As theory does not exist in isolation, a second method of verification is to look for similar findings in related literature. Such a search, while demonstrating that the research is unique, will demonstrate how the new work fits in to what is already known in a field.

Theoretical verification

First, verification of findings with participants is an important step in the research process. When verifying a study, the investigator must be cautious in presenting the findings to ensure that the research does not ask leading questions and thus force verification. One important strategy is to present the entire model or theory to the participants and then ask for a response. To ask the participants to verify the theory by asking low-level, closed-end questions provides the participants with the right answer, the desirable answer, thus invalidating the validation procedures.

Second, verification with related literature is important. No study exists in isolation, independent of the work of others. Research must be embedded in the conceptual world, as well as in the research context. For theoretical evaluation, the researcher must identify related concepts found in similar settings. For example if the researcher is studying caring, the results must at least in part be identified in the work of other researchers when investigating similar topics.

ISSUES OF RIGOUR

Rigour in any research is required to prevent error of either a constant or intermittent nature. Initially, qualitative research work was criticized because empirical researchers believed there was a lack of control over the validity and reliability of the findings. Since then, attention has been paid to the need to develop trustworthiness in qualitative research.

One of the earliest attempts to address this issue was made by Lincoln and Guba (1985) who described four general criteria for the evaluation of qualitative research, defining each criterion from both a qualitative and quantitative perspective. Lincoln and Guba's model addresses four aspects of trustworthiness that they believed to be relevant to both quantitative and qualitative studies. They called these **truth value, applicability, consistency** and **neutrality**.

Truth value or credibility Truth value is subject-oriented and not defined in advance by the researcher. Lincoln and Guba (1985) used the term **credibility** which they related to internal validity in empirical research. In empirical research the assumption is made that there is only one tangible reality to be measured. In qualitative research one recognizes that there are multiple realities, so the researcher's job becomes one of reporting the perspectives of the informants as clearly as possible.

Applicability Applicability is the criterion used to determine whether the findings can be applied in other contexts or settings or with other groups. Lincoln and Guba (1985) note that in the quantitative perspective applicability refers to how well the threats to external validity have been managed.

Consistency Consistency is the third criterion used to evaluate trustworthiness. Here the emphasis is on whether the findings would be consistent if the inquiry were replicated with the same subjects or in a similar context. In quantitative research the concern is with the extent to which an instrument will provide the same measurement over time. In field research, where one assumes multiple realities, the notion of reliability is no longer as relevant. Qualitative research emphasizes the uniqueness of the human situation, so that variation in experience rather than identical repetition is to be expected.

Neutrality or confirmability Another criterion used to establish rigour is freedom from bias in the research procedure and results. In empirical research, objectivity is the criterion of neutrality and is achieved through the rigour of methodology by which reliability and validity are established. Qualitative researchers try to increase trustworthiness by prolonged contact with the informants or by using long periods of observation. Researchers also try to identify their own biases through the use of memos and through consultation with other researchers.

The audit trail

Recently, emphasis has been placed on the development of an audit trail to clearly document researcher decisions, choices and insights. Such a trail is clearly described by Rodgers and Cowles (1993) who identify areas where documentation should occur. They note the importance of ordered and dated field-notes to place interviews within context. For example if an informant cries, this may indicate an emotional part of an interview, but tears may be evident before crying becomes audible on a tape. Changes in methodological approach, with the rationale, need to be noted in a diary or in memos. For example the focus of interview questions may change as themes or concepts begin to emerge from the data. It is important to be able to report at what time and for what reason the changes occurred.

It is critical that the researcher find a system of recording that is personally acceptable. When recording, be descriptive; record first, then discuss with friends and colleagues, and always synchronize your notes with other data. Also, record your subjective interpretations of events to keep you alert to areas of potential bias.

Areas of concern for reliability and validity

LeCompte and Goetz (1982) addressed the issues of reliability and validity in ethnographic research, identifying some critical areas where error can occur. They identified five areas where external reliability could be affected: the status position of the researcher; informant choices; the social context in which data are gathered; the definitions and delineations of the constructs and their relationships; and the methods of data gathering and analysis. LeCompte and Goetz (1982) argue that the strength of qualitative research is high validity. This is not always the case. Research which is based on single interviews with an individual or in which information has been withheld due to lack of credibility of the researcher with the informant will not be valid. Participant observation can enhance validity, but there is also the risk that the researcher may go native and lose objectivity. Internal validity basically addresses the problem of whether conceptual categories have shared meaning between the participants and the researcher. Phenomena can change over time. Factors which can create change include the history and maturation of the group, the selection of informants, mortality from the study and spurious conclusions.

External validity

Threats to external validity are those effects that obstruct or reduce a study's comparability. Four factors have been identified by LeCompte and Goetz (1982) that might affect the credibility of groups across situations: selection effects, setting effects, history effects and construct effects.

Leininger (1994) also addresses the issues of credibility (truth value, believ-ability). She argues that the major threat to credibility is too little time in the field to understand the lived-through experiences of those studied. To ensure confirmability the researcher must obtain evidence from informants on the researcher's findings or interpretations, returning to the informants to check the emerging theory. Leininger also recommends the use of audit trails and triangulation of data sources. Leininger also cautions that one must under-stand data within a holistic context, which includes actions, events, commu-nication and other relevant contextual and environmental factors. It is critical to look for patterns of events or repeated experiences rather than single, albeit spectacular, occurrences. Saturation refers, in Leininger's explication, to the need to undertake an exhaustive exploration of the phenomena under study. Her final criterion is that of transferability, i.e. whether there are general similarities which can be applied under similar conditions, contexts or circum-stances.

External validity is enhanced by synthesizing the results of studies that examine the same phenomena but in different contexts and then comparing and contrasting the results. An example of this is The Illness-Constellation Model (Morse and Johnson, 1991, pp. 315–42). In this chapter, the results of five studies, conducted in a variety of situations in which individuals were diagnosed with and treated for an illness, are synthesized and the overall process of responding to illness identified. In this way, qualitative contribu-tions contribute substantially to mid-range theory development (See Aggre-gating research findings, Chapter 7).

Further issues

In 1986, Sandelowski described the problem of rigour in qualitative research and the use of Lincoln's and Guba's (1985) criteria rather than the inappro-priate use of the terms **reliability** and **validity**. More recently, Sandelowski (1993) has moved away from her initial position, believing that there is an inflexibility and an uncompromising harshness and rigidity implied in the term **rigour** that take us too far from the 'artfulness, versatility and sensitivity to meaning and context that mark qualitative works of distinction' (p. 1). Fur-ther, she sees one of the major threats to constructing validity (the views of the informants) as the assumption that validity rests on reliability. She also argues that repeatability is not an essential property of qualitative interviews or qualitative research. Sandelowski's (1993) comments outline the difficulty of arriving at one set of criteria for qualitative research when in fact it encom-passes a wide range of approaches and methods. While Sandelowski believes member validation may be a threat to validity rather than a safeguard when both member and researcher are stakeholders in the research process, others would disagree. Further, she identifies similar problems in relation to valida-tion measures such as peer debriefing and triangulation, where convergence may be inappropriately sought. Her warning is that the measures taken to safeguard trustworthiness are complex and that the researcher must examine them carefully before selecting those that are appropriate to the research in hand.

PRINCIPLES

- Qualitative analysis is an active process which requires the researcher to become immersed in and have complete familiarity with the data.
- Four cognitive processes are integral to all qualitative analysis: compreheading, synthesizing (decontextualizing), theorizing, and recontextualizing.
- Data collection and analysis occur simultaneously. As interviews are transcribed, checked and corrected, coding begins.
- Field-notes are written (or dictated), typed into the computer and analysed along with the interviews.
- Coding can be done by hand or by using a program for textual analysis; the method selected depends on the researcher's style and the amount of data.
- Approaches to content analysis will depend on the method selected: latent and manifest content analysis or by stages and phases.
- Categories and themes generally arise from the data and are labelled as themes emerge across interviews.
- Tentative propositions (hypotheses) about relationships within the data will develop as relationships begin to emerge among behaviours, participants' activities and so forth.
- Issues in qualitative research relate to subjectivity, the quality of the evidence presented by the researcher and whether or not interpretations have been validated with participants.
- Issues of rigour include truth value, applicability, consistency and neutrality.
- An audit trail should be maintained to document the researcher's decisions, choices and insights, and to assist the researcher in demonstrating theoretical rigour.

REFERENCES

Atkinson, P. (1990) *The Ethnographic Imagination: Textual Constructions of Reality*, Routledge, New York.
Babbie, E. (1979) *The Practice of Social Research*, 3rd edn, Wadsworth, Belmont, CA.
Denzin, N.K. (1978) *Sociological Methods: A Sourcebook*, 2nd edn, McGraw-Hill, New York.
Field, P.A. (1984) Behaviour and nursing care, in *Care: The Essence of Nursing and Health*, (ed. M. Leininger), J.B. Slack, New Jersey, pp. 249–62.

Fox, D.J. (1982) *Fundamentals of Research in Nursing*, 4th edn, Appleton-Century-Crofts, Norwalk, CT.

Glaser, B.G. (1979) *Theoretical Sensitivity*, The Sociology Press, Mill Valley, CA.

Heider, K. (1983) The Rashomon effect. *Association for Social Anthropology in Oceania Newsletter*, Spring issues, pp. 10–11.

LeCompte, M.D. and Goetz, J.P. (1982) Problems of reliability and validity in ethnographic research. *Review of Educational Research*, **52**, 31–60.

Leininger, M. (1994) Evaluation criteria and critique of qualitative research studies, in *Critical Issues in Qualitative Health Research Methods*, (ed. J.M. Morse), Sage, Thousand Oaks, CA, pp. 95–115.

Lincoln, Y.S. and Guba, E. (1985) *Naturalistic Inquiry*, Beverly Hills, Sage.

Lofland, J. (1971) *Analyzing Social Settings: A Guide to Qualitative Observation and Analysis*, Wadsworth, Belmont, CA.

Miles, M.B. and Humberman, A.M. (1994) *Qualitative Data Analysis*, Sage, Thousand Oaks, CA.

Morse, J.M. (1991) Analyzing unstructured, interactive interviews using the Macintosh™ computer. *Qualitative Health Research*, **1**(1), 117–22.

Morse, J.M. (1991/92) Negotiating commitment and involvement in the patient — nurse relationship, in *Qualitative Health Research*, (ed. J.M. Morse), Sage, Newbury Park, pp. 333–59.

Morse, J.M. (1992) If you believe in theories... (editorial). *Qualitative Health Research*, **2**(3), 259–61.

Morse, J.M. (1994) 'Emerging from the data': the cognitive processes of analysis in qualitative inquiry, in *Critical Issues in Qualitative Research Methods*, (ed. J.M. Morse), Sage, Melno Park, CA, pp. 23–43.

Morse, J.M. and Bottorff, J.L. (1989) Intending to breast-feed and work. *Journal of Obstetrical, Gynecological and Neonatal Nursing*, **18**(6), 493–500.

Morse J.M. and Johnson, J.L. (eds) (1991) *The Illness Experience: Dimensions of Suffering*, Sage, Newbury Park, CA.

Rodgers, B.L. and Cowles, K.V. (1993) The qualitative research audit trail: a complex collection of documentation. *Research in Nursing and Health*, **16**, 219–26.

Sandelowski, M. (1993) Rigor or rigor mortis: the problem of rigor in qualitative research revisited. *Advances in Nursing Science*, **16**, 1–8.

Spradley, J.P. (1980) *Participant Observation*, Holt, Rinehart and Winston, New York.

Tripp-Reimer, T. and Cohen, M.Z. (1991) Funding strategies for qualitative research, in *Qualitative Nursing Research: A Contemporary Dialogue*, rev. edn (ed. J.M. Morse), Sage, Newbury Park, CA, pp. 243–57.

Weitzman, E. and Miles, M.B. (1995) *Computer Programs for Qualitative Analysis*, Sage, Newbury Park, CA.

FURTHER READING

Atkinson, P. (1992) *Understanding Ethnographic Texts*, Sage, Newbury Park, CA.

Ball, M.S. and Smith, G.W.H. (1992) *Analyzing Visual Data*, Sage, Newbury Park, CA.

Denzin, N.K. (1989) *Interpretive Interactionism*, Sage, Newbury Park, CA.

DeWalt, B.R. and Pelto, P.J. (eds) (1985) *Micro and Macro Levels of Analysis in Anthropology*, Westview, Boulder, CO.

Feldman, M.S. (1995) *Strategies for Interpreting Qualitative Data*, Sage, Thousand Oaks, CA.

Fielding, N.G. and Fielding, J.L. (1986) *Linking Data*, Sage, Beverly Hills, CA.

Fielding, N.G. and Lee, R.M. (1991) *Using Computers in Qualitative Research*, Sage, London.

Gubrium, J. (1988) *Analyzing Field Reality*, Sage, Newbury Park, CA.

Kirk, J. and Miller, M.L. (1986) *Reliability and Validity in Qualitative Research*, Sage, Beverly Hills, CA.

Miles, M.B. and Huberman, A.M. (1994) *Qualitative Data Analysis*, 2nd edn, Sage, Newbury Park, CA.

Pfaffenberger, B. (1988) *Microcomputer Applications in Qualitative Research*, Sage, Newbury Park, CA.

Psathas, G. (1995) *Conversation Analysis: The Study of Talk-in-Interaction*, Sage, Thousand Oaks, CA.

Riessman, C.K. (1993) *Narrative Analysis*, Sage, Newbury Park, CA.

Rosengren, K.E. (1981) *Advances in Content Analysis*, Sage, Beverly Hills, CA.

Silverman, D. (1993) *Interpreting Qualitative Data*, Sage, London.

| 7 | **Qualitative approaches** |

In this chapter selected qualitative methods introduced in Chapter 2 will be discussed in greater depth. These methods include phenomenology, grounded theory, ethnography and ethnoscience. Issues in conducting qualitative research will then be examined, such as rigour, reliability and validity. Finally, techniques of triangulation will be described and methods of synthesizing qualitative studies will be presented.

PHENOMENOLOGY

Phenomenology is not just a research method but also a philosophy and an approach. In phenomenology the researcher seeks a deeper and fuller meaning of the experience of the participants of a particular phenomenon. Phenomenology offers a descriptive, reflective, interpretative and engaged mode of inquiry (van Manen, 1990). Wilson and Hutchinson (1991) note that phenomenological researchers do not talk about a 'method' *per se*, but rather 'discuss the tradition, the reading, reflection, and writing process' that enables the researcher to 'transform the lived experience into a textual expression of its essence' (van Manen, 1990). Phenomenologists try to describe the experience as it is and to describe it directly without the various causal explanations. For example when reading Clarke's (1990/92) 'Memories of breathing: a phenomenological dialogue: asthma as a way of becoming', the reader can identify with the mother and the daughter's experiences of managing asthma. The reader does not have to be an asthmatic to be able to sense the essence of breathlessness, the mother's concern and her daughter's attempts to 'not panic' (i.e. to appear normal) and devise ways to take her breathalyser inconspicuously in the presence of her peers.

The foundations of phenomenology are rooted in the work of the German philosopher, Husserl. His work was carried on by Heidegger who described the basic structure of the life world, focusing on the **lived experience**. Experience is considered as one's perceptions of one's presence in the world at the moment when things, truths or values are constituted. The four existentials that guide phenomenological reflection are **lived space (spatiality), lived body (corporeality), lived time (temporality), and lived human relation (relationality or communality)** (van Manen, 1990). Perceptions present us with evidence of the world, not as it is thought but as it is lived. For example if one considers 'lived space', a mother would look at a kitchen cupboard and say, 'It is 8 feet tall, I must get a ladder'. Yet a cat's perception of that space is that it is a sink and a refrigerator away. Our perception of space differs because of our different experience.

Another assumption of phenomenologists is that human existence is meaningful and of interest only in the sense that we are always conscious of something. Existence as 'being in the world' is a phenomenological phrase that acknowledges that people are tied to their worlds (embodied) and are understandable only in their contexts. Human behaviour occurs in the context of relationships to things, people, events and situations.

A phenomenologist may argue that we see the world as an already-interpreted phenomenon, that is as the result of past scientific inquiry. For example we are limited in what we see. In phenomenology we try to understand how people **attend** to the world, remembering that in all individual description there is also interpretation (Boyd, 1993; van Manen, 1990).

In phenomenological conversation, the interview is presuppositionless. Ray (1994) notes that the research questions are not predetermined, but rather 'flow with a clue-and-clue-taking process' (p. 129). In order to grasp an essence, concrete experiences are considered and then the researcher tries to imagine that experience, modifying it by trying to imagine it from all aspects. The purpose of this reflection is to find out what is essential in order for the phenomenon to be. To achieve this, phenomenologists use a wide variety of resources to find the essence of meaning. They engage in conversations with others, obtain descriptions from the literature and poetry, watch films and reflect on the phenomenological literature.

Spielberg, cited in Boyd (1993), describes seven steps in arriving at essence. The first is **intuitive**, which involves developing one's consciousness through looking and listening. This is followed by **analysing**, which involves identifying the structure of the phenomenon under study and which occurs through dialectic (the conversation between participant and researcher). This knowledge is created through a joint project in which respondent and researchers are jointly committed to describing the phenomenon under study. The third phase is **describing the phenomenon**; however, premature description is one of the potential dangers in phenomenology. Description directs the listener to explore his/her own experience of the phenomenon. Insight becomes communicated through description. The next two steps involve **watching modes of appearing** and **exploring the phenomenon in consciousness**. At this stage the researcher reflects on the relationships (or structural affinities) of the phenomenon. For example consider the relationship between pain and hurt. The researcher will look to see under what conditions pain is experienced (modes of appearing),and the nature and the meaning of pain. The final two stages are **suspending belief** (phenomenological reduction) and **interpreting concealed meanings**. This latter step is used in hermeneutic phenomenology to describe the lived experience in a way that can be of value in informing our practice and science.

Insights into the phenomenon are gained using a number of techniques: tracing etymological sources, searching idiomatic phrases, obtaining experiential descriptions from a respondent and observing and reflecting further on the phenomenological literature and writing and rewriting (van Manen, 1990; Ray, 1994). In analysis, words or phrases that describe some aspect of the lived experience are listed separately from each other. Similar expressions are grouped and labelled. Irrelevant expressions are eliminated. Then groups of expressions that bear close relationships to one another are clustered and labelled. The identified core of common elements is checked against a selection of original descriptors obtained in conversations with the respondents. Discrepancies direct the researcher to revisit the analysis.

Different schools use different terminology and approaches to analysis. Van Manen (1990) and Benner (1994) talk more of ordering of themes and of acquiring an intuitive grasp of the textual data. While these differences can be attributed to the fact that phenomenological method has evolved in more than one direction with interpretative (hermeneutic) phenomenology, all phenomenologists subscribe to the belief that 'human being is a unique way of being in that human experience and actions follow from their self-interpretation' (Benner, 1994, p. ix).

The best way to learn to appreciate phenomenology is to read it. In addition to Clarke's (1990/92) 'Memories of breathing', examples of phenomenological studies are Kelpin's (1984/92) 'Birthing pain' and Smith's (1989/92) 'Operating on a child's heart'. The journal, *Phenomenology + Pedagogy*, has many excellent examples.

ETHNOGRAPHY

When doing ethnography, the researcher seeks to understand the cultural perspective of the group using participant observation, interviewing and field-notes. Boyle (1994) notes that ethnography is always holistic, contextual, reflexive and is presented from the emic perspective. To study a culture, the researcher must spend time in the field (Fetterman, 1989).

A classical ethnography must include both a description of behaviour and demonstrate why and under what circumstances the behaviour took place. Fieldwork is essential in ethnographic research and involves working with people for long periods of time in the naturalistic setting. The researcher is both a participant in and an observer of the group that is being studied. One cannot develop a cultural understanding or the emic perspective through only one or two interviews; time in the culture is essential to obtain a holistic perspective.

In the health sciences, a more delineated (yet still context-bound) ethnography has evolved, known as **focused ethnography** (Morse, 1987; Muecke, 1994). Muecke notes that focused ethnographies are used primarily to improve practice and differ in important dimensions from the classical ethnography. For instance the topic is selected before data collection commences, rather than emerging during data collection and analysis. While participants are linked by a common site, this location may be a treatment site (such as a clinic) rather than a place of residence. Participants may not be connected by the same culture (in its broadest sense), but share behavioural norms and a common language emanating from experiencing a common illness. Participant observation is limited to particular events or times, and interviews are generally limited to the selected topic and surrounding event.

The techniques for data collection (for both classical and focused ethnography) include interviews and observations, recorded as field-notes and documenting everyday events. Sampling includes both individuals in the culture and events which occur within the group that adds to the researcher's understanding of the values and norms. Description of the context in which the behaviour occurs is a critical dimension of an ethnographic study.

Examples of focused ethnography include Cassell's (1987/92) work on surgeons, Golander's (1987/92) description of nursing home residents, and Rosenham's (1973/92) study of psychiatric patients. An example of focused ethnography is Field's (1984) description of community health nurses. Boyle (1994) notes that there are many variations of ethnography, suggesting that while ethnography is a method, 'an ethnography' is also the end product of that method.

The earlier discussions on gaining entry and finding key informants are particularly relevant in ethnography. One must establish rapport, become comfortable in the setting, and become familiar with the custom and nuances of language used in the particular setting. Establishing credibility and trust are critical if the researcher is to obtain relevant and adequate data. Again, participants are selected on the basis of their knowledge of the culture and their willingness to talk about the event.

Data collection and analysis take place concurrently. The researcher may need to learn about the group's history, religion, politics, economy, environment, and about special subgroups within the culture. Obtaining these data is labour intensive as it involves prolonged and direct contact with the group.

The first phase of analysis involves understanding essential cultural schemas (Agar, 1986). The ethnographer, in attempting to understand a culture, develops a schema about how behaviour is patterned. When behaviour does not comply with expected behaviour, the strip 'breaks down' and must be resolved. The resolution process involves the repeated application of 'strips to schemas', by modifying and reapplying the schema to the strip until a coherent explanation is derived (Agar, 1986). Agar also notes that the sequential resolution of schemas pushes the analysis to a greater level of abstraction until cultural patterns are realized.

Most ethnographers use direct quotations from the informants that summarize or illustrate the concept or theme being described. Analysis involves reading each interview or set of field-notes for themes and examining relationships between themes. Researchers identify the values and rules that govern behaviour in the group and examine their influence on group cohesion and norms. As the research develops, the questions move from broad general questions, such as 'Tell me about...', to contrast questions (e.g. 'How is health promotion different from health prevention?'), or to questions which seek out similarities and differences between properties or attributes of a concept.

Descriptive ethnography will identify the social complexity that underlies the society. However, most ethnographies reveal more depth as the researcher explains social patterns or observes conduct that may not be evident even to members of the cultural group. Thus, thick description (Gertz, 1973) permits the development of interpretative or analytic ethnography (Turner and Bruner, 1986). Ethnographers do not take data at face value but regard them as inferences from which cultural patterns may be identified and tested (Boyle, 1994). The end product should inform the reader about the normative behavioural patterns of the group studied.

GROUNDED THEORY

The term **grounded theory** is used in relation to a particular form of data collection and analysis. It was developed by two sociologists, Glaser and Strauss (1967) who were, at that time, members of the Chicago School of Sociology. They developed both a new philosophical approach and method to identify basic social processes within the context in which these processes occurred.

The underlying principles of grounded theory were derived from the Chicago School (Strauss) and Columbia University (Glaser). Strauss was influenced by the writings of social interactionists (such as Everett Hughes and Herbert Blumer) and the pragmatists (who included Robert Park and John Dewey). Glaser was influenced by Paul Lazanfeld, who was an early innovator in the use of qualitative methods in sociology. The goals of both Strauss and Glaser were to produce research that would be of value to professional and lay audiences, and to develop solid theory that fitted with reality.

The primary purpose of grounded theory is to generate explanatory models of human behaviour which are grounded in the data. Data collection and analysis of data occur simultaneously. The generation of the theory is based on comparative analyses between or among groups within a substantive area using methods of field research for data collection. Using grounded theory, a researcher seeks to identify patterns and relationships between these patterns (Glaser, 1978; 1992). For example as no work had been done on attaching behaviours of mothers of preterm infants, grounded theory was used to look at these particular mothers (Brady-Fryer, 1994) and a theory of 'Becoming a mother to a preterm infant' emerged. The data obtained provided a tentative theory from interviews and observations in the naturalistic setting.

Grounded theory is non-linear in nature and hence is difficult to describe. The process is both hierarchical and recursive, as researchers must systematically categorize data and limit theorizing until patterns in the data emerge from the categorizing operation. This method requires data collection, open categorising, memoing, determination of a core category, recycling of earlier steps in terms of the core category, sorting of memos and the write-up of the theory.

The data collection and analyses are closely linked at every step of the way. To meet the four central criteria of fit, work, relevance and modifiability (Glaser, 1992), theoretical sampling is also employed. This entails finding informants or events to assist in fleshing out thin areas of data as the theory emerges. This sampling is not predetermined but ongoing, dependent on the needs evidenced in the emerging theory. If grounded theory is done well, the reader will find explanations about observed behaviours comprehensive, inductively tied to the data with emerging hypotheses that are both appropriate and plausible.

When using a grounded theory approach, the researcher must consider several factors. The setting itself influences the way in which behaviour is evidenced and therefore it must be taken into consideration in data analyses. There must be an adequate range of participants to provide a full range of variations in the phenomenon so that definitions and meanings are grounded in the data. If the participants are restricted to an homogeneous group, this fact must be made clear. The descriptions of social behaviours should be as they occur in their natural settings, which means that, in interviews, the researcher must also ask questions that identify the 'what' and the 'where' of each described situation. All behaviours must be understood from the participant's perspective. This takes skill, as the researcher must be both participant and observer in the participant's world in order to reach this level of understanding.

It is difficult to be very specific about a problem until data collection is under way. The researcher goes into the field to make observations that may be of assistance in categorizing or explaining a phenomenon, thus generating theory and concepts associated with it.

The researcher must make a conscious effort to eliminate preconceived beliefs about the phenomenon under study, and the purpose is to allow the data to dictate identification of concepts, linkages and ultimately grounded theory uncontaminated by the researcher's personal biases and prejudices. For example Brady-Fryer (1994) went into the field to study attaching behaviours of mothers of preterm infants, only to find that the basic social concern was how to mother an infant that was in the preterm nursery. As a consequence, research questions may change as the study progresses and as they become influenced by the data collection and analysis process. A researcher must enter the field with a focus and be able to justify the relevance of the study, but be open and sensitive to initial data which lead to an identification of a basic social problem.

Theoretical sampling

Theoretical sampling in grounded theory is the process of data collection for generating theory, whereby the analyst jointly collects, codes and analyses data and decides what data to collect in order to develop a theory as it emerges (Glaser, 1978). Thus the data collection process is influenced by the outcomes of the emerging analysis. It proceeds through successive stages, which are determined by changes in the criteria for selecting interviewees according to what has been learned from previous data sources. Participants are therefore chosen as needed rather than before the research begins.

Data analysis

The constant comparative method of data collection and analysis is used in grounded theory, that is each piece of data is compared with every other piece of relevant data. Data derived from interviews and observations may be summarized by the researcher from field-notes or verbatim transcriptions from tape recordings. All relevant concepts are identified and codes are assigned to each piece of data.

Glaser and Strauss (1967) write of using 'constant comparison' during this phase of analysis. This means that the data must be examined closely for all instances of phenomena that seem to be similar, whether or not there is a fit with the developing category. For example if one has three interviews with one individual, comparison of data across all three interviews would be required to identify all examples of the category of person, behaviour or event being labelled or saturated. Comparisons should also be made across interviews provided by different informants. A category is said to be saturated when no new information on the characteristics of the category is forthcoming.

First level coding

During this process, all interview transcripts are analysed line by line, and descriptive code names are written in the right-hand margin. These codes apply to phrases, sentences or groups of sentences within the data that represent common concepts. At this stage, a descriptive label is attached to each concept described by the participant. Each incident in the data is coded into as many codes as possible to ensure full theoretical coverage, so as to allow the emerging theory to fit the data and explain the behavioural variations. It is possible for one sentence to have more than one assigned code or, at times, two or three sentences are combined to form one code.

The first level of coding is called **substantive** or **open coding** (Glaser, 1978). Action words (gerunds) ending in 'ing', such as crying, singing and laughing, are used. The researcher restates the facts as closely as possible to the participant's words or documented observed phenomena characteristics. Open codes are clustered, based on similarity or dissimilarity of content. The primary purpose is to elucidate the theoretical properties of each category. Open coding comes to an end when a core category is identified. Since this type of coding is based on facts, it limits the imposition of the researcher's biases.

As the researcher codes the information, ideas, insights, thoughts and feelings about the relationships in the emerging theory are documented in the form of memos which serve the following functions:

- help the research to obtain insight into tacit, guiding assumptions;
- increase the conceptual level of the research by encouraging the researcher to think beyond single incidents and look for themes and patterns in the data;
- capture speculations about the properties of the categories or relationships among categories, or possible criteria for selection of additional partici-pants to enrich the data;
- enable the researcher to keep track of and preserve ideas that may be potentially valuable later in the study but which may be premature at this stage in the study;
- are important in noting thoughts about similarity of emerging theory to established theories and concepts.

It should be noted that memos are written about other memos. These memos are sorted and compared as the theory becomes more streamlined. If at any stage the researcher is not sure whether or not his/her biases are affecting the perceptions of the phenomenon, then observations should be augmented with informal or semi-formal interviews to clarify perceptions and 'ground' the data.

Selective coding

The second step in the coding process is to categorize, recategorize, and condense all the first level codes, ensuring that all the concepts remain un-changed, unless they become irrelevant as more incoming data are analysed and interpreted. The goal is to identify the relationships of the dimensions or properties of the categories. Categorizing moves the coding process to a higher level of abstraction. The basis of the coding scheme is constantly reviewed to determine validity and reliability.

Once concepts which show some relatedness are identified, the literature is reviewed to help generate further questions and research problems. As this circular process continues, some concepts being to appear more prominent than others. Interconnections between the categories begin to emerge as certain patterns and linkages are identified. Some basic properties start to define themselves as 'certain differences between incidents create boundaries and relationships between categories are clarified' (Hutchinson, 1986, p. 118). This type of coding is called **axial** (Corbin and Strauss, 1990).

The next task is to review the analytical documentation and sort the memos in order to summarize the theoretical explanations. The researcher searches for saturation of content where only a few new incidents may be added to the categories that will demonstrate a new dimension to the problem. At this stage, all levels of codes will yield no new information, all variables and behaviours are accounted for, and the researcher gets a feeling of completeness. Saturation is reached when no new information is identified which would indicate that new categories were emerging or that old codes needed expanding.

After saturation has been achieved, the researcher summarizes the theoretical explanations, after making further comparisons with the existing literature. The question of what constitutes the basic social problem is examined. This is followed closely by a second question which explores the basic social process (BSP) which helps the participants to cope with the problem (Hutchinson, 1986). It is the core category which assists with the emergence of the BSP. The BSP must explain all variations in the problem being studied, predict behaviours, and show how these processes may evolve over time. With the 'fixing' of the theory, the report is ready to be written.

The emergence of hypothetical relationships represents the beginning of theory emergence. As the interrelationships become more apparent, the core categories begin to become evident, and other categories combine and change position in the emerging structure. Once the core category has been identified, the core variable then becomes a guide to further data collection and theoretical sampling. Codes, memos and integration start occurring in relationship to the core variable (Glaser, 1978). In the analytic process of delineating the stages and characteristics of each stage, diagramming and mapping the relationships between variables clarifies and enables increased level of abstractness to be obtained.

One strategy of diagramming is the construction of typologies (Glaser, 1978). The researcher first identifies two variables or emerging concepts that appear to contribute to the variance in the phenomenon and, using a 2×2 matrix, explores the effects of the presence or absence of each variable in the four combinations. Finally, diagrams or models of the process or sequence assist to illustrate the relationships of the various concepts or the process of moving through the various stages and phases of the experience.

It should be remembered that theoretical sensitivity — the ability of the researcher to recognize what is important in the data and to give it meaning — is absolutely essential in grounded theory. It helps to formulate theory that is faithful to the reality of the phenomena under study. Theoretical sensitivity comes from continual interaction with the data through collection and analysis and by being well-grounded in the technical literature. If the researcher is sceptical and uses constant comparisons, data contamination will be avoided and theoretical sensitivity will be achieved.

Additional examples of grounded theory are Morse and Bottorff (1988/92) 'The emotional experience of breast expression', Morse and Johnson (1991) *The Illness Experience: Dimensions of Suffering* and Field and Marck (1994) *Uncertain Motherhood: Negotiating Risk in the Childbearing Years*.

ETHNOSCIENCE

In ethnoscience, data are collected through a series of tape-recorded interviews. To ensure adequate depth of understanding, a minimum of three interviews is necessary with each informant. The data are transcribed and analysed between interviews.

Defining the domain

At the first interview, broad questions that clearly define the domain are asked. For example if the topic is 'difficult patients', broad questions may be, 'Have you ever nursed difficult patients?', 'What kinds of "difficult" patients are there?', and 'What are the different ways nurses manage "difficult" patients?' Listen very carefully for lexemes, labels used by the group; in this case, the words nurses use to describe the patients. For instance nurses may describe 'difficult' patients as 'naughty', 'noisy', or 'bossy', 'attention seeking', or as 'a wanderer'. As these types of difficult patients form the basis for each contrast set in the analysis, it is important to transcribe and list these lexemes.

Sentence frames

At the second interview, the attributes of each type of difficult patient are obtained, firstly, with the use of open-ended questions contrasting two different types of patients. For instance the researcher may ask, 'What is the difference between an "attention-seeking" patient and a "demanding" patient?' Secondly, sentence frames confirm the unique characteristics of each contrast set, and should be used both with the same informant and other informants. Sentence frames are essentially statements which ask the respondent to fill in the blanks. For example:

A_____ patient_____
    (type)   (action)

The respondent might complete the sentence as follows:

A **demanding** patient **rings the bell too often**.

Card sorts

Finally, the commonalties between the different types of components are established by the use of dyadic and triadic card sorts and the Q-sort. The interviewer writes all the attributes of each component on separate cards and, for the dyadic card sort, asks the informants to sort the cards into two piles. When the informant has finished, the researcher asks the informant to name each pile and to describe the differences. For example the informant may have sorted patient characteristics into two piles, one labelled 'bossy' and the second labelled 'demanding'. The informant is then asked to sort the cards into three piles and to describe and label each pile. This increases the information obtained by the researcher. Some behaviours will remain in the 'bossy' and 'demanding' piles. Behaviours common to both sets of patients may be in the third pile.

In the Q-sort, the informant is given the cards to sort into piles. The number of piles is not forced by the researcher but determined by the informant. Again, when the task is finished, information concerning the differences and commonalties between each pile is elicited from the informant by the researcher.

Preparation of a taxonomy

From the segregates and sub-segregates it is possible to sort the categories into a taxonomy. Although there are several styles or methods of presenting the data, the principles are the same. The researcher will now need to search further to determine whether the characteristics are unique to each category and whether further characteristics can be identified related to each classification.

Taxonomies may also be developed that relate to events rather than to people. An example of this would be a taxonomy relating to decision making in childbirth. The first part of the taxonomy may be related to who makes decisions, while the second part identifies the types of decisions that are made by each category of person involved in the process. To develop this second taxonomy, the researcher needs to ask structural questions. In this instance information would need to be elicited to determine what types of decisions the informants think they can make in the specified situations. One can ask 'What are the different kinds of decisions you can make about labour?' and 'What are the different ways in which you participated in making decisions?' In asking structural questions, one can go from specific to general or general to specific.

Some propositions can be formulated into this taxonomy. These might be related to which participants make decisions during labour and the dimensions in which the various participants hold power to determine the outcome.

The researcher might wish to learn the attributes of a particular category. For example 'doctor' is a perceptual category, but there are certain structural components that can be identified that further classify the abstract concept. There are types of doctors, with various levels of expertise and experience. A structural question may be, 'What are the different kinds of doctors you encounter in the hospital?' An attribute question, to get more specific responses, could be phrased, 'What is the difference between a general practitioner and a resident?' (or any other paired category). In this manner, named categories and their attributes can be developed.

Examples of ethnoscience are Spradley's (1984/92) 'Beating the drunk charge' and Morse's (1991a) 'The structure and function of gift-giving in the patient–nurse relationship.'

METHODOLOGICAL TRIANGULATION

Is it possible to use both qualitative and quantitative methods in the same study? The answer is most definitely 'yes', and often the strongest research findings are in studies that utilize both methods. Multiple methods of data collection enrich the perspectives that the researcher has on the phenomenon. The mix can occur either sequentially or simultaneously, and may combine either two qualitative methods or a qualitative and a quantitative method. The study design is dependent on the theoretical drive of the project (Morse, 1991b).

Sequential

Qualitative and quantitative methods may be used sequentially as the project develops, with qualitative methods used initially until the hypotheses emerge. At this stage hypotheses may be tested using appropriate quantitative methods on a larger sample. For example when examining parturition pain in the Fijian and Fiji-Indian women, Morse (1989) used ethnographic interviews to understand the cultural context of childbirth. Then, to confirm hypotheses regarding differences in the amount of pain attributed to childbirth in each culture, the expected painfulness of parturition was measured using a psychological scale.

Simultaneous

Qualitative and quantitative methods may be used simultaneously to address the same problem. This technique is known as **triangulation** (Jick, 1979). Qualitative methods may be used to describe the affective aspects of the domain, while quantitative methods may be used to measure other variables. A questionnaire, for example may contain both standardized psychological tests in addition to open-ended questions that must be analysed qualitatively and that will permit more freedom in the individual's response. Morse and Doan (1987) used this technique when examining adolescents' response to menarche. Open-ended, short-answer questions were used to elicit information on the girls' feelings towards their first period. However, the same 'test-package' contained a Likert scale to measure attitudes toward menstruation and psychological tests such as draw-a-person.

Another way in which qualitative and quantitative methods may be used together is when the researcher wishes to use a quantitative research design using qualitative measurement. This is useful when some of the variables may not be suitable for quantification. For example a researcher may wish to examine the effect of preparing parents for their child's surgery and measure the effectiveness of their care by using proxemic (spatial distance) behaviour as the independent variable. The hypothesis may be that, by encouraging parents to move close and comfort the child, despite the child's condition and the presence of equipment, the child will be less anxious postoperatively. As proxemic behaviour is a variable that is difficult to quantify, a qualitative measurement of parent–child personal space may be used in conjunction with other quantitative measures.

Wilson and Hutchinson (1991) describe the use of two qualitative methods to enhance the researcher's understanding of the phenomenon. They illustrate their article by triangulating Heideggerian hermeneutics and grounded theory, and argue that, while each method has its own integrity and produces different outcomes, triangulation of the results of these studies 'can illuminate clinical realities that elude alternative approaches'. In the proposal (Appendix A), three qualitative methods are triangulated to understand the construct of comfort: phenomenology, grounded theory and ethnoscience. Phenomenology was used to determine the meaning of comfort; grounded theory, the process of providing comfort; and ethnoscience, the components of comfort. Note that as the interviewing techniques are different, each of these data sets — and the analysis — are kept separate until each study is complete. It is the **results**, not the data, that are triangulated.

SYNTHESIZING QUALITATIVE STUDIES

As findings from qualitative studies begin to appear with greater frequency, it is important to consider examining them for similarities and differences. It is suggested that findings from independent but similar research may be aggregated with a cohesive study (Estabrooks, Field, and Morse, 1994). Analysis and synthesis of findings from several studies will increase the level of abstraction and lead to greater generalizability.

In the approach advocated by these authors, the individual undertaking the analysis and synthesis does not return to the original data but uses the findings presented by the original researcher. This differs from approaches identified by Thorne (1994), which include analytic sampling, armchair induction, amplified sampling and cross-validation. All these approaches require either amplification or re-analysis of the original data.

In discussing synthesis of studies, the work by Noblit and Hare (1988) must be considered. They use the term **aggregate** to denote a context-stripping activity rather than an interpretive one. In Noblit and Hare's discussion, the goal of meta-ethnography was comparison and synthesis rather than theory development. A recent example of meta-ethnography is the work by Jensen and Allen (1994) in which they undertake a synthesis of qualitative research describing the illness experience.

In synthesizing findings, it is important to select studies that focus on similar populations and themes. It is also advisable to select studies that use similar research methods. The third criterion is that themes reported by the original researchers must be clearly labelled and rooted in the data. While categories may not always have been given the same labels across studies, common themes will emerge if the original labels are clearly rooted in the data. This type of analysis should not be undertaken by a novice researcher. The work is conceptually demanding and requires considerable skill in interpretation to aggregate findings.

PRINCIPLES

- Common qualitative designs include case studies, one group and two group design, and triangulation of qualitative and qualitative–quantitative methods.
- The type of triangulation used depends on the theoretical drive (quantitative or qualitative) of the study.
- Phenomenology is used when the researcher wishes to describe the essence of the experience.
- Ethnography is used for describing phenomena within the cultural context.
- Grounded theory is used to describe a process, and to develop mid-range explanatory theory.
- The purpose of ethnoscience is to identify and document the cognitive domain or perception of phenomenon.
- Synthesis of findings across independent, qualitative research that addresses a common topic may lead to the development of rigorous theory.

REFERENCES

Agar, M.H. (1986) *Speaking of Ethnography*, Sage, Beverly Hills, CA.

Benner, P. (ed.) (1994) *Interpretive Phenomenology*, Sage, Thousand Oaks, CA.

Boyd, C.O. (1993) Phenomenology: the method, in *Nursing Research: A Qualitative Perspective*, 2nd edn, (eds P.L. Munhall and C.O. Boyd), National League for Nursing, New York, pp. 99–132.

Boyle, J.S. (1994) Styles of ethnography, in *Critical Issues in Qualitative Research Methods*, (ed. J.M. Morse), Sage, Thousand Oaks, CA, pp. 159–85.

Brady-Fryer, B. (1994) Becoming the mother of a preterm baby, in *Uncertain Motherhood*, (eds P.A. Field and P.B. Marck), Sage, Thousand Oaks, CA, pp. 195–222.

Cassell, J. (1987/92) On control, certitude, and the 'paranoia' of surgeons, in *Qualitative Health Research*, (ed. J.M. Morse), Sage, Newbury Park, CA, pp. 170–91.

Clarke, M. (1990/92) Memories of breathing: a phenomenological dialogue: asthma a way of becoming, in *Qualitative Health Research*, (ed. J.M. Morse), Sage, Newbury Park, CA, pp. 123–40.

Corbin, J. and Strauss, A.L. (1990) *Basics of Qualitative Research: Grounded Theory Procedures and Techniques*, Sage, Thousand Oaks, CA.

Estabrooks, C., Field, P.A. and Morse, J.M. (1994) Aggregating qualitative findings: an approach and theory development. *Qualitative Health Research*, **4**, 503–11.

Fetterman, D.M. (1989) *Ethnography: Step by Step*, Sage, Newbury Park, CA.

Field, P.A. (1984) Behaviour and nursing care, in *Care: The Essence of Nursing and Health*, (ed. M. Leininger), J.B. Slack, New Jersey, pp. 249–62.

Field, P.A. and Marck, P.B. (1994) *Uncertain Motherhood: Negotiating Risk in the Childbearing Years*, Sage, Thousand Oaks, CA.

Gertz, C. (1973) *The Interpretation of Cultures*, Basic Books, New York.

Glaser, B.G. (1978) *Theoretical Sensitivity: Advances in the Methodology of Grounded Theory*, The Sociology Press, Mill Valley, CA.

Glaser, B.G. (1992) *Emergence Versus Forcing: Basics of Grounded Theory Analysis*, The Sociology Press, Mill Valley, CA.

Glaser, B.G. and Strauss, A.L. (1967) *The Discovery of Grounded Theory: Strategies for Qualitative Research*, Alden, Chicago.

Golander (1987/92) Under the guise of passivity, in *Qualitative Health Research*, (ed. J.M. Morse), Sage, Newbury Park, CA, pp. 192–201.

Hutchinson, M. (1986) Grounded theory: the method, in *Nursing Research — A Qualitative Perspective*, (eds P. Munhall and C. Oiler), Appleton-Century-Crofts, Norwalk, CT, pp. 111–30.

Jensen, L. and Allen, M. (1994) A synthesis of qualitative research on wellness – illness. *Qualitative Health Research*, **4**, 349–69.

Jick, T.D. (1979) Mixing qualitative and quantitative methods: triangulation in action. *Administrative Science Quarterly*, **24**, 602–11.

Kelpin, V. (1984/92) Birthing pain, in *Qualitative Health Research*, (ed. J.M. Morse), Sage, Newbury Park, CA, pp. 93–103.

Muecke, M.A. (1994) On the evaluation of ethnographies, in *Critical Issues in Qualitative Research Methods*, (ed. J.M. Morse), Sage, Thousand Oaks, CA, pp. 187–209.

Morse, J.M. (1987) Qualitative nursing research: a free-for-all? in *Qualitative Nursing Research: A Contempory Dialogue*, (ed. J.M. Morse), Sage, Newbury Park, CA, pp. 14–22.

Morse, J.M. (1989) Cultural responses to parturition: childbirth in Fiji. *Medical Anthropology*, **12**(1), 35–44.

Morse, J.M. (1991a) The structure and function of gift-giving in the patient–nurse relationship, in *Qualitative Health Research*, (ed. J.M. Morse), Sage, Newbury Park, CA, pp. 236–58.

Morse, J.M. (1991b) Approaches to qualitative – quantitative methodological triangulation. *Nursing Research*, **40**(1), 120–3.

Morse, J.M. and Bottorff, J.L. (1988/92) The emotional experience of breast expression, in *Qualitative Health Research*, (ed. J.M. Morse), Sage, Thousand Oaks, CA, pp. 319–32.

Morse, J.M. and Doan, H.M. (1987) Adolescents' response to menarche. *Journal of School Health*, **57**(9), 385–9.

Morse, J.M. and Johnson, J.L. (eds) (1991) *The Illness Experience: Dimensions of Suffering*, Sage, Newbury Park, CA.

Noblit, G.W. and Hare, R.D. (1988) *Meta-ethnography: Synthesizing Qualitative Studies*, Sage, Newbury Park, CA.

Ray, M.A. (1994) The richness of phenomenology: philosophic, theoretic, and methodologic concerns, in *Critical Issues in Qualitative Research Methods*, (ed. J.M. Morse), Sage, Thousand Oaks, CA, pp. 117–33.

Rosenham, D.L. (1973/92) On being sane in insane places, in *Qualitative Health Research*, (ed. J.M. Morse), Sage, Newbury Park, CA, pp. 202–24.

Smith, S. (1989/92) Operating on a child's heart: a paedological view, in *Qualitative Health Research*, (ed. J.M. Morse), Sage, Newbury Park, CA, pp. 104–22.

Spradley, J.P. (1984/92) Beating the drunk charge. *Qualitative Health Research*, (ed. J.M. Morse), Sage, Newbury park, CA, pp. 227–35.

Thorne, S. (1994) Secondary analysis in qualitative research: issues and implications, in *Critical Issues in Qualitative Research Methods*, (ed. J.M. Morse), Sage, Thousand Oaks, CA, pp. 263–79.

Turner, V.W. and Bruner, E.M. (1986) *The Anthropology of Experience*, University of Illinois Press, Urbana, IL.

van Manen, M. (1990) *Researching Lived Experience: Human Science for an Action Sensitive Pedagogy*, Althouse, London, Ontario, p.10.

Wilson, H.S. and Hutchinson, S.A. (1991) Triangulation of qualitative methods: Heideggerian hermeneutics and grounded theory. *Qualitative Health Research*, **1**(2), 263–76.

FURTHER READING

Bogdan, R.C. and Biklen, S.K. (1982) *Qualitative Research for Education: An Introduction to Theory and Models*, Allyn and Bacon, Boston.

Chenitz, W.C. and Swanson, J.M. (1986) *From Practice to Grounded Theory*, Addison-Wesley, Menlo Park, CA.

Clough, P.T. (1992) *The End(s) of Ethnography: From Realism to Social Criticism*, Sage, Newbury Park, CA.

Hammersley, M. and Atkinson, P. (1983) *Ethnography: Principles in Practice*, Tavistock, London.

Heritage, J. (1984) *Garfinkel and Ethnomethodology*, Polity Press, Cambridge.

Jorgensen, D.L. (1989) *Participant Observation: A Methodology for Human Studies*, Sage, Newbury Park, CA.

Miles, M.B. and Huberman, A.M. (1984) *Qualitative Data Analysis: A Sourcebook of New Methods*, Sage, Beverly Hills, CA.

Moustakas, C. (1990) *Heuristic Research: Design, Methodology, and Applications*, Sage, Newbury Park, CA.

Moustakas, C. (1994) *Phenomenological Research Methods*, Sage, Thousand Oaks, CA.

Noblit, G.W. and Engel, J.D. (1991/92) The holistic injunction: an ideal and a moral imperative for qualitative research, in *Qualitative Health Research*, (ed. J.M. Morse), Sage, Newbury Park, CA, pp. 43–9.

Sandelowski, M. (1986) The problem of rigor in qualitative research. *Advances in Nursing Science*, **8**, 27–37.

Sandelowski, M. (1993) Rigor or rigor mortis: the problem of rigor in qualitative research revisited. *Advances in Nursing Science*, **16**, 1–8.

Shafer, R.J. (1980) *A Guide to Historical Method*, 3rd edn, Wadsworth, Belmont, CA.

Spradley, J.P. (1980) *Participant Observation*, Holt, Rinehart and Winston, New York.

Sproull, L.E. and Sproull, R.F. (1982) Managing and analyzing behavioral records: explanations in non-numeric data analysis. *Human Organization*, **41**, 283–90.

Stern, P.N. (1980) Grounded theory methodology: its uses and processes. *Image*, **12**(11), 20–3.

Stern, P.N., Allen, L.M. and Moxley, P.A. (1984) Qualitative research: the nurse as grounded theorist. *Health Care for Women International*, **5**, 371–85 (original work published 1982).

Turner, B. (1981) Some practical aspects of qualitative data analysis: one way of organizing the cognitive processes associated with the generation of grounded theory. *Quality and Quantity*, **15**, 225–47.

Werner, O. and Schoepfle, G.M. (1987a) *Systematic Fieldwork: Foundations of Ethnography and Interviewing*, Vol. 1, Sage, Newbury Park, CA.

Werner, O. and Schoepfle, G.M. (1987b) *Systematic Fieldwork: Ethnographic Analysis and Data Management*, Vol. 2, Sage, Newbury Park, CA.

Wolcott, H. (1975) Criteria for an ethnographic approach to research in schools. *Human Organization*, **34**, 111–28.

Zelditch, M. Jr. (1969) Some methodological problems of field studies, in *Issues in Participant Observation: A Text and Reader*, (eds B.J. McCall and J.L. Simmons), Addison-Wesley, Menlo Park, CA, pp. 5–19.

Reporting qualitative research | 8

The purpose of doing any research is to **answer a question**. The completed research should advance knowledge and therefore be of interest to the scientific community. As the questions to be answered in applied sciences are often derived from the clinical setting, the final phase of the research process is the application and evaluation of the research. Therefore, unless the results are written up **and published**, they cannot fulfil any useful purpose, and the effort in conducting the research is for nought. These issues are, of course, in addition to any personal gain that the researcher may have as a student, which is the completion of requirements for a degree or a personal contractual obligation to a funding agency that has supported the research. Besides, it is thrilling to be able to contribute in a small way to the development of knowledge: to provide information for teachers to teach, for researchers to build on, for clinicians to use and to improve patient care. This is only possible if the results are disseminated.

In this chapter, the process of writing for publication will be addressed, with some hints about how to overcome common problems and pitfalls when writing. Next, methods of evaluating a qualitative report as a reader and as a researcher wishing to build on the findings, will be presented. Finally, a means for evaluating a qualitative report for the possible utilization of the findings will be discussed.

WRITING QUALITATIVE RESEARCH

The purpose of conducting research is to add to the knowledge base underlying the discipline, and perhaps to impact on and improve clinical practice. This cannot occur unless the research results are published and, if the results are not published, all the effort and expense of conducting research is wasted. There is no doubt that the researcher has not completed the research process until the report, thesis or dissertation has been published. In this chapter, the process of writing qualitative research will be examined: for whom to write and how to write the article. Next, suggestions for presenting qualitative findings, including poster and oral presentations, will be discussed. Criteria for evaluating qualitative articles will be presented and, finally, how to consider utilizing qualitative findings in the clinical setting.

Getting started

The first step in writing an article is to clearly identify what you have to say, and to whom you wish to say it. Therefore, the first task is to be certain about the purpose and content of the article. Identify an audience and select the journal in which you wish the article to appear. As journals are particular not only about the bibliographical style, but also about the style of writing and how the article is written, this decision must be made before the writing begins if extensive rewriting is to be avoided.

Other things must be ready before beginning to write. The analysis must be finished. Even though the researcher may be writing intensely throughout the process of data analysis — and some of those notes may be incorporated into the text with minor editing — the theoretical work of the research must be completed. Otherwise, how would the researcher know what to write in the article? Yet beginning the manuscript too early is a common error. Therefore, firstly, outline the article, select the quotations that may be included and prepare any tables or figures necessary.

For whom to write? All writing is basically a political process, whether to debunk or modify the present status quo, to add to or enhance someone else's work, to synthesize and clarify current knowledge or to present methodological or clinical innovation. Each of these categories is generally met by specialist journals, all with varying degrees of receptivity to qualitative research. But it is the researcher's responsibility to select the right journal to reach the right readership, and the writing study should be a reasonable fit with other articles published in the selected journal. Another piece of advice is that a smart researcher does not expect to have work accepted in the first journal to which it is submitted. Normally the article will be rejected; otherwise a revision may be requested. A request for a revision is good news, for articles are rarely accepted without changes.

Writing qualitatively

The nature of qualitative research and the fact that data are descriptive and stored and retrieved as text lulls the researcher into false expectations that, after months of 'writing it down', 'writing it up' will be the easiest part of the research process. But there are traps that catch the unwary — writer's block that impedes the process, the effort of having abstracts using less than mainstream methods accepted for conferences, and the difficulties of publishing qualitative findings cause unexpected frustrations and delays. The delays and problems of disseminating qualitative research often threaten to quench the effectiveness of months of work.

Writer's block

Some time ago, Morse received an invitation to serve as a consultant for a post-doctoral programme. 'Our qualitative researchers,' she was told, 'are having trouble writing up their data.' Despite the fact that qualitative researchers may deliberately select the level of abstraction to which they push their analysis, and some researchers intentionally leave their results at the descriptive level, the qualitative researcher **does not write up data**. Perhaps this impression is fostered because the most descriptive qualitative reporting appears to consist simply of quotations linked together with minimal textual commentary. However, this is not the case: it is the **analysis** that is reported, not the data, and until the analysis is completed, how will the researcher know what to write? Perhaps the greatest cause of writer's block is premature writing, with the researcher attempting to write before the analysis is completed, before the emergent theory is polished and connected with the work of others, or even before the analyst has thought through **what he or she wants to write**.

Besides 'thinking an article through' before beginning to write, the researcher may find that presenting or explaining the content to colleagues is very helpful. Somehow, putting the thoughts to words facilitates the process of putting the words on to paper. Furthermore, the questions that arise from the discussion assist the researcher to see any gaps or conceptual leaps that have been made where his or her reasoning is not quite clear. The process of explaining the results and responding to questions helps to clarify the model for the researcher. Also, assuming that 'two (plus) heads are better than one', the theoretical knowledge of these colleagues may provide other conceptual linkages for the researcher that increase the theoretical generalizability of the study, making the research stronger and more significant than the researcher previously realized. These colleagues may be experts in qualitative methods or know nothing of the methods and assumptions; they may be familiar with the topic or it may be unfamiliar; they may be clinical experts in the area or know little about the application — for the most fruitful discussion, a mixed seminar is best.

The nuances of qualitative writing

The general goal in qualitative writing is to present the data so that the reader shares the participants' experiences. The quotations serve to put the 'the voices in the text', while vivid description leads to synthesis, and combines with contextual data to develop theoretical formulation.

However, there are many nuances to writing qualitatively. Qualitative researchers use quotation marks frequently in their writing to draw the reader's attention when a common word is being used uncommonly. The quotation marks may indicate that the word was used deliberately to denote that the word is being used as it is used by participants or to denote the special meaning intended. The latter case Minnich (1990, p. xvi) refers to as 'scare quotes' to indicate that the words are being used deliberately, 'self-consciously', where she uses the language for the reader to hear 'as it vibrates between levels and across situations and realms of meaning'. This particular use of quotations is problematic for copy editors who are unfamiliar with qualitative work, and may not recognize their significance.

Editing participants' quotes

During the transcription process, it is important that all of the interview material be transcribed verbatim, that pauses be indicated and that all expressions be included in the text. While these directives are important for maintaining the integrity of the data during the analysis phase (for it enables the researcher to continue to 'hear' the interview), to place unedited transcription directly into the document adds nothing to the reader's appreciation of the results. In fact, the opposite occurs. Rather than illustrating a particular point and making the researcher's message clearer, the unedited quote will distract the reader, and the message that the researcher is trying to convey will be obscured by the irrelevant material. In fact, the quotations may be so difficult to read that the reader may skip them altogether.

The next question is how to cull the quotations and still maintain the integrity of the data? Conventions of standard punctuation usually are sufficient to indicate to the reader that editing has taken place (Field and Morse, 1985). For example if only a part of the quotation is needed, and the first part of the paragraph is excluded, replace the first part of the paragraph with three ellipsis points (i.e ....). Similarly, if an irrelevant sentence is removed from the middle of a paragraph, replace this with four ellipsis points to signal to the reader that the text has been cut. A pause may be indicated with a long dash (—) while a thoughtful, lengthy pause may be inserted into the text in square brackets: [long pause]. Any emotional reactions that are necessary to include may be inserted inside square brackets: [laughs] or [crying]. In addition, square brackets may be used to indicate who is being referred to when the person's name is removed, thus: J_____ [brother]. If participants use grammatical errors when speaking, these should remain in the quote but be acknowledged with a [*sic*]. Accents are more difficult to transcribe, and should be transcribed with care to avoid insulting the ethnic group whose dialect is being phonetically written. Furthermore, as will be discussed later in maintaining anonymity, if only one of the participants in the setting has an accent, then adding this characteristic to the quotation will clarify the speaker of those words to all those familiar with the setting and who read the publication, thus violating the researcher's agreement to conceal participants' identity.

Maintaining anonymity

One important task in writing qualitative research is to maintain the anonymity of all agreements made at the time the research was negotiated. This includes not revealing the identity of the participants and the research site — including the institution and, frequently, even the location or city in which the research was conducted.

Note that this section is addressing only **anonymity**. In qualitative research, if you intend to quote the participant's words, confidentiality cannot be ensured and consent forms should make this clear. Suggested wording could be:

> Our interviews will be tape-recorded and these will be transcribed without anyone's name. Following our interview, our conversation will be transcribed, but your name will not be on the transcription associated with the study, or on any publication resulting from this research, although some of your words may be included in these reports.

However, despite the fact that **names** are removed from all quotations, the inclusion of tags and other identifiers may enable those who know who participated in the research — including participants themselves — to indirectly link identifiers and thus reconstruct the informant's identity. The more tags or links left by the investigator, the easier this process may be, and the greater the risks for the participants when the report is disseminated.

Therefore, it is recommended that as few as possible identifiers be placed in the report. Strategies that may be used include the following.

- Report only aggregate demographic information, such as ages in ranges and so forth. Even if the numbers of participants are fewer than 10, do **not** prepare a table that lists each person by age, marital status, gender, ethnicity and so forth. Determining those who participated in the study and who did not is only a matter of elimination for those familiar with the research setting.
- Do not place an identifier at the end of each quote, even if it is a pseudonym. Often quotes may be linked to a participant by a single comment, and such a clue would then enable someone to link and pool all quotations published from that person's interviews.
- If it is important to place some identifiers at the end of each quotation, such as age and gender of the participant, then it is permissible to systematically change the ages of all participants by a few years, just as it is permissible to provide pseudonyms or to change the names of cities to protect the participants. But remember to alert the reader in a footnote to the fact that the actual names/ages/locations have been changed in the report.

It is important to note that, in qualitative research, the sample probably was not selected to participate in the study because of particular demographic characteristics, but rather because of some other life experience. For example a researcher studying experiences of SCI (spinal cord injury) patients and coping may need to interview patients who have remained hopeful and who have coped well on discharge, and others who did not. These characteristics would therefore determine the selection of participants, rather than age, gender and so forth. Glaser (1978) notes that demographic characteristics should not be considered significant until they emerge as significant and earn their way into the emerging model. Our compulsion to report these factors may be inherited from our quantitative colleagues and may jeopardize our sample and yet have little to do with the ability to replicate the study or the sample. Finally, it is wise to have the article or report read carefully by a colleague to ensure that anonymity has been maintained.

Reporting negative findings to the 'host'

One of the most difficult tasks in writing qualitative results — and one that can be so problematic that writing becomes impossible — is to maintain validity, to remain, as Bergum (1989/91) describes it, 'true to your data' and to include the negative, uncomplimentary, **critical** things from your data in the final report. A problem arises when these results have to be reported back to the agency or institution where the study was conducted, there they may not be received graciously by (or may even offend) those who so willingly permitted the researcher access. While it is immoral and against research ethics not to report problems the study revealed, by reporting them, the researcher risks alienating his or her 'host'.

The first task is to prevent the **fear of offending** from looming so large as to prevent anything from being written at all. Write the first draft as well as you can, with descriptive fairness that does all your research skill justice. Then explain your dilemma to a colleague, whose judgment you trust, and ask that person to read this draft, flagging anything that may be offensive or problematic. It is possible that you, as researcher, are simply being overly sensitive to the whole matter and few, if any, changes will be required. If changes are required, perhaps it will be possible to write the critical portions more softly or with more justification, so that the conclusions are evident. Or, place all the negative comments in the quotations, so that the document reads as if the participants are speaking. And if the worst comes to the worst, consult with a lawyer before releasing the findings. However, there is no guarantee that this will prevent problems, such as the subpoena of data to 'confirm the findings' that Barinaga's (1992) report on DiFranza and his colleagues' research on 'Old Joe Camel' recently revealed.

Another strategy may be to present a trusted contact in the host organization with the negative findings to 'test the waters'. It is possible that the organization may be aware of the problem (but not the underlying cause) and grateful for the information. Alternatively, that person may be able to diffuse the findings at the board meeting where the results are to be presented, so that the raw truth does not appear so shocking. When presenting, the use of the royal 'we' (by including oneself, as a fellow professional, or as a fellow human stuck in the same dilemma, the same world and so forth) will soften the blow and help develop a more constructive atmosphere towards the results. If there is absolutely no way around the problem, take a colleague with you when you present — someone to pick up the pieces, buy you a drink and drive you home.

Building a case

There are two basic styles of presenting qualitative work. The first is to present a synopsis, or overview of the resulting theory to serve as a road map for the reader, and then to follow these paragraphs with the supporting data. The second style is to present the results as the project was conducted, so that the reader shares the insights and the conclusion that the researcher gained, bit by bit and step by step. In both cases, by the time the reader has reached the end of the results sections, they will share the researcher's conclusions.

The researcher's conclusions should be clear, with alternative explanations and hypotheses systematically excluded, and with in-depth descriptions that vividly portray each point. Examples — informant quotes, exemplars and case histories — added judiciously provide richness. Subheadings should be used to keep the reader on track and to highlight each point.

Using quotes

The effective use of quotes is important in the research. The participant's quotes should only be used when the participant has made a point in a manner better than the researcher could make by himself/herself. Except in the case of presenting unwelcome results (as previously mentioned), the point that the researcher is trying to make should be clearly described in the few paragraphs before the quote is used. In this case, the quote illustrates the paragraph. The full range of diversity, or the characteristics and the synthesis of all the material pertaining to that section, should be included in the text: remember that the quotes **supplement** the text and provide human insight and dimension to the analysis. As previously mentioned, the quote may be edited and the extraneous material removed from the segment.

One of the most common mistakes made by new researchers is that they consider almost **all** of their data significant and **all** of their quotes vital. Removing any of the quotes by even hinting that they are repetitive, redundant or insufficiently important is met with a storm of protest, heart rending exclamations of pain and threats of suicide. Remember: it is easier to be tough on yourself than to be torn to shreds by another.

Diagramming, modelling and the use of tables

The presentation of some qualitative methods is particularly enhanced by the use of diagramming, modelling or the effective use of tables to provide overviews or schemes of the study. They serve to keep the reader on track and often attract the attention of the casual person flipping through the journal. They may even be useful for the researcher: diagrams, figures and tables should be prepared first — while the article is being outlined — and may, therefore, even assist the research in the process of writing by preventing derailments or diversions to less significant material.

Grounded theory is particularly suited to diagramming, as the end product is substantive or formal theory (Chenitz and Swanson, 1986). The stages, phases and strategies of each part may be listed in a summary, or the model may be diagrammed with the direction and processes of the **BSP (Basic social process)** or the **BSPP (Basic social psychological process)** explicated with arrows (Morse and Johnson, 1991). Ethnography is also often easily diagrammed with the characteristics of each category listed in a table (such as the taxonomies of ethnoscience in Spradley and McCurdy, 1972).

GETTING PUBLISHED

Books and monographs

Qualitative research is best disseminated as book length manuscripts, as this gives the research enough space to **really** tell the reader what it was like. However, publishing books has several disadvantages. Often, books do not have the rigorous review that an article undergoes and, therefore, are not as highly regarded in some universities as a refereed article. Secondly, they are not accessed as easily as articles through such bibliographical retrieval services as *Medline*, where one can locate an article by author, title or topic and obtain a copy of the abstract on-line. Advantages are tremendous, however; the main one being that once a contract is obtained, the publication of the book is more or less assured. Not only that: a year or two after publication, royalties may even be possible.

Obtaining a contract

It is prudent to approach several publishers to determine their preliminary interest in publishing your manuscript. Invariably, the publishers will ask for your proposal, so have this ready to send out. Rather than submitting this to one publisher (as in the case of an article), a proposal may and should be sent to many publishers simultaneously.

The editor will provide you with the instructions for preparing a proposal. Basically, the proposal will consist of the titles and a few paragraphs about the book. A Table of Contents is welcome. The proposal should have a few paragraphs about you as an author, stating your writing experience, why the book is unique, what its competing volumes are and why you are qualified to write the book. Attach some completed chapters and a sample of the book and your writing. The publisher will copy many of these proposals and send them to experts nationwide to review and comment on.

Publishing articles

To split or not to split

Frequently, the first decision to be made when preparing an article for publication, is to delineate the content of the article: where to 'split' the report or dissertation in order to divide it into publishable, manageable units. The skill is to maintain significant content and focus in the articles, **with rigour and richness**, without 'overdiluting' or making the report into too many articles so that none of them have adequate theory or substance to stand alone. There is often pressure on more junior faculty members to err on the side of more publications, since, in the 'publish or perish' context, **numbers of articles** (rather than important, fewer and more substantive articles) are valued for achieving tenure and promotion. Yet, journal editors are suspicious of articles that refer to several others that appear similar — editors are afraid of copyright violation and prefer to publish **really** original work. Even if the author goes on to write several articles around the first one published, editors realize that subsequent articles must cite or otherwise acknowledge the first article, and such citations will enhance subscription rates.

Presenting papers at conferences will assist the researcher in identifying units of interest to colleagues, and will provide some 'feel' for whether or not the units will be able to stand alone from the questions and the response of the audience. It is wise to deliberately plan the content of each paper, rather than to let papers simply 'emerge'. Often, the order in which the articles are submitted for publication is important; essential papers may then be referred to as 'in press'.

Identifying the audience

The 'audience' or journal readership is most important to consider before submitting an article, for the targeted readership will determine the focus of the article. Is the article to be written for researchers or clinicians? If readers are experienced researchers, they will not require much in-depth explanation of the method; if they are neophyte researchers, they may be as interested in **how to do the research** and demand a clear and detailed explanation. Does the clinical audience primarily consist of doctors, nurses and other health professionals, or a mixture of health care professionals? If the readership is clinical, are the **implications for practice** clearly written, along with any caveats or concerns?

Choosing the journal

Some journal editors have implemented regulations that weaken the reporting of qualitative research. Most commonly, editors' insistence on restricting the length of submissions to 15 pages (and often fewer) make it difficult for qualitative researchers, because rarely can all the requirements for the richness of description be developed in a short article. Other editors may insist that a certain outline be strictly adhered to for acceptance, and this outline may not be conducive to the presentation of qualitative reporting. For example the insistence that a literature review must be presented before the results may not be ideal for a study using grounded theory, when linkage to the literature is inherent within the presentation of results. Van Manen (1990) notes that presentation of a research question and description of the method is not necessary for phenomenology — such sections make for an unnecessary distraction from the poetics of the writing. Another case may be made for describing the method only when it deviates from a standard description that is more clearly presented in a methodology text. For instance reading summary after similar summary of grounded theory in article after article is really unnecessary, when the reader could easily be referred to Strauss (1978) or Strauss and Corbin (1990). Space in our journals is too expensive for such luxuries, and the same standards of explication are not required of quantitative researchers. As May (1989/91) notes, quantitative researchers may briefly describe their method and provide a citation, and these same standards should be acceptable for qualitative researchers.

When to submit?

One of the most difficult decisions for a new researcher is to recognize when an article is actually finished and polished enough to submit. It is recommended that when you think the article is finished, put it away and read it after a day or two. Read it out loud. Does the article say what you intended? Or has your thinking matured and is another draft necessary?

A smart researcher never sends an article to a publisher without both a peer review (for content) and an editor's check (for style and format). The fresh eyes, sharp eyes, will spot areas of weakness, omissions and other problems in the manuscript that were previously hidden and would have been embarrassing if they had gone out without being corrected. Check the article for consistency. Does the title match the purpose and fit what the article is about? Does the abstract provide a fair description? Does the conclusion actually conclude the article or does it leave the reader 'dangling'? Check the article for 'balance' — the literature review should not overshadow the results section, since it is the results that are of greatest interest to the reader. Finally, check the format, making sure that the editorial specifications of the journal are met. Please do not 'trick' the system by shortening the article by reducing the font size and the margins. Such strategies do not reduce the length of the published article, and it is the number of printed pages that are of concern to the editor. Finally, ensure that all the bibliographical entries are correct and comma perfect.

Adhering to format

Format is important. Meeting format requirements is really a technical task. Nevertheless a correct format is important, and if it is neglected or unsatisfactory, then the article will be sent back to the author for correction and may even not make it to press.

One of the most common and careless errors is that authors do not send all their pages to the editor or may even leave out a figure. This problem may occur during copying or may be a word processor error. Occasionally the editor notices and can fax for the missing page; or, more often, the reviewer notes it and the whole process of review is delayed while the reviewer notifies the editor, who notifies the author, who mails it to the editor, who mails it to the reviewers, who then continue with the review ...

A second problem is the author's use of a dot matrix printer to print the final versions. Dot matrix does not copy well, especially if the ribbon is not new. A smart researcher uses a laser printer, even if it means a trip to a laser print shop. Reviewers must be able to **read** what they are evaluating. Similarly, most journals require that the document be **double-spaced** to give the editor room to work; to add, delete and alter the text. **Everything** must be double-spaced, including quotes and the references.

Checking the reference list for completeness is vital. Most journals restrict the reference list to those sources cited, and, for space reasons, some even restrict the number of citations. It is most important that the format of the references matches that requested by the journal, for the typesetters will type what they see. If the format differs from the journal's own format, the editor can only conclude that the article must have been rejected from another journal and the author did not even bother to disguise this fact by changing the style. The editor will then be in a mind-set to 'find the error' when reading it, and then, perhaps unfairly, assume that there must be some fatal flaw in the manuscript.

Finally, when submitting (and only to one journal, please), ensure that the requested number of copies are submitted. Editors get grumpy if they have to dash to the machine and duplicate, because they feel they have more to do with their time and the department's funding. When the article is ready to go, slide it into the postbox with a wish and a prayer — not forgetting, of course, to watch for an acknowledgment of the receipt of the article and to inquire after its status if too many months go by.

Managing editors

'I like what you say, but hate the way you write.' Unfortunately, most editors have their own pet peeves and their own preferred style. Sometimes editors are 'up front' with these quirks and will list them in their style sheets. Other times authors may discover them serendipitously, by attending a workshop or meeting authors who have previously published in that journal. At other times authors may discover these preferences the hard way, by submitting and receiving back their edited manuscript.

What are these fads of editors? They may be minor and not affect the submission if the author is prepared to revise (for example a title consisting of a colon and a subtitle, or the use of the passive voice). In this case, editors will specifically inform you how to fix the article. Other times these preferences may result in major revisions or rejection of the article. Of importance are authors who will not consider qualitative studies, perhaps because they do not understand qualitative methods or do not consider qualitative research rigourous or a science. When selecting a journal, look back on previous issues to see how the articles are directed, how they are presented and if qualitative research has been published in that journal.

Responding to reviewers

One of the more delicate tasks of the editor is to serve as a mediator between the reviewers and the author, to evaluate the reviewers' remarks and to make a decision of whether to accept, reject or to request revisions on an article. The editor may summarize the comments and give very clear directive to the author, or the editor may forward all the comments to the author. In the latter case, some of the reviewers remarks/criticisms may be contradictory. One reviewer may write complimentary remarks about a particular passage; a second reviewer may pull it to 'shreds' and request it to be revised.

Should the author be caught between two conflicting positions, the onus is on the author to respond either by revising the article or by responding to the editor in a covering letter ('I concur with Reviewer A and have not altered the third paragraph; Reviewer B is not apparently familiar with methods for selecting qualitative samples.') Remember, the author is responsible for the content of the article — and a part of this responsibility is to write clearly. It is important, therefore, that if some passage is unclear, the author should take negative criticisms very seriously and try to understand why a certain point was unclear or misinterpreted.

ORAL PRESENTATIONS

On the surface, presenting qualitative research should be easier than quantitative findings. Qualitative findings are not hampered with tables consisting of numbers of graphs, charts and figures. Qualitative research should lend itself naturally to 'story telling', to verbal presentation.

Unfortunately, this is not always the case. First, there is rarely enough time in a 15-minute presentation to present a comprehensive, **complete** study. Thus, the researcher is forced to artificially focus and present one narrow portion of the study. Invariably, a member of the audience will ask, 'What about ...', and the researcher will predictably explain, 'Well, I do have that included in my model, but there was not enough time to discuss it.'

Second, presenting qualitative studies **in depth** necessarily requires more time than a quantitative study. Qualitative data cannot be presented as neatly and as efficiently in quantitative tables and figures. In order to present the qualitative data, the context must be described, the participants' experiences explained and quotes read and the emerging theory explicated. Slides or overheads do much to facilitate this process and help the listener to grasp the main points. If participants' quotes are placed on the slide, the listener can read the words with the presenter, which may add even more meaning to the presentation. Well done, qualitative presentations may be profoundly moving.

PREPARING EFFECTIVE POSTERS

Qualitative results take up more space than a quantitative summary because the context is more significant than who the subjects were. Therefore, when preparing a poster, the qualitative researcher should primarily present the findings. Depending on the qualitative methods used in the project, emphasize the categories developed and the relationships between them. Diagram models. Photographs really catch the attention of the audience: a picture is worth a thousand words.

VIDEOS

As a means of presenting qualitative research, videos may be the most powerful technique: the viewer can see and understand the setting and the experience as the researcher sees it. However, to summarize research results as a documentary complete with commentary is extraordinarily expensive and a most time-consuming endeavour.

An alternative may be to use the video to **illustrate** the presentation and for the researcher to provide the commentary — the interpretation or analysis — over the audio portion or by turning the sound off. This technique provides the researcher with greater versatility with the video, since the portions of video may be selected and substituted as the focus of the presentation changes.

Timing of the video segments and the presentation is important, with the researcher practising to ensure that the presentation will not extend beyond the allocated time. Once the presenter has begun the presentation, the time is 'fixed' and cannot be hurried or truncated — only terminated if the chair decides that time is 'up'.

EVALUATING QUALITATIVE RESEARCH

Compared with quantitative research, qualitative research has relative absence of standards for evaluation. Whereas quantitative researchers have clear guidelines for determining the adequacy of the sample, in qualitative research saturation is used as an indicator of sampling adequacy, and this is, in part, a decision of the investigator, evidenced by the absence of 'thinness' in the data presented and the richness of descriptions as evidenced in the text. Qualitative research does not have the convenience of clear p values and other statistical indicators, as quick indicators of the significance of the research. However, even though the process is more complex than quantitative research, the task is necessary and important for the continued construction of a solid foundation for the profession and for the evolution of clinical practice. In this section, first the process of assessing the significance of the research report or article. Note that this process of assessing the worth of the **article** is different from a **research audit** (Rodgers and Cowles, 1993), in which the auditor evaluated the research process, reconstructing the process of inquiry, including examining raw data.

Evaluating the significance of the research

All research begins with a question, although the question may not be explicitly stated in all qualitative research. Van Manen (1990) writes that to state directly a question **as a question** is unnecessary in phenomenological research, where the purpose is to engage the reader into the experience. However, regardless of whether or not the question is directly stated or implied, research, whether qualitative or quantitative, **must be worth the effort**. It must extend knowledge, provide new insights — adding to or refuting theory or revealing new areas of investigation. While qualitative methods are not usually used to confirm or to replicate findings, the results should fit into the work of others. Thus, the researcher normally will have made a case for conducting the research at the beginning of the article or report, and, in the discussion will have stated what the contribution of the study is and why it was important. If the article does not contain any new or unique information, that is if it does not make a contribution, then the article is of dubious value.

Theoretical evaluation

The level of the theoretical development of a qualitative article depends on the type of qualitative method used and the purpose of the study. An article, such as narrative inquiry reporting on data obtained from a single case, should be more than the editing and presentation of the transcripts. The article must reveal the intellectual work of the investigator, and this process is independent of the number of participants in the study. For example a 'case study' using narrative inquiry may reveal the theoretical development of the article in a number of ways. For instance in one study, Morse and Carter(1995), after introducing the study, presented the participant's narration. The second part of the article is a commentary on the transcript; the third, theoretical development of the data; and, finally, the discussion section links the emerging theory with other literature. In sum, the researcher, even with case study interview data, must be more than an editor of an audiotaped story.

Some qualitative methods lend themselves to developing theory more than others. The strength of grounded theory is that it is well-suited to developing models and mid-range theory. Excellent theory also may be obtained by using ethnography or ethnoscience, whereas a phenomenological study may make a descriptive contribution, sensitizing the reader to the human experience and adding to the phenomenological perspective of temporality, spaciality, relationality and corporeality (van Manen, 1990).

Methods used to evaluate theory have been well described (Glaser, 1978). First, assess the level of abstraction to determine the explanatory power of the theory. As stated, minimally, qualitative research should add insight and perspective. But the qualitative study could also suggest theory that may be implemented (refer to the next section on using qualitative findings), be tested, organize diverse observations and identify and develop concepts.

The presentation of the findings must contain adequate description for the reader to follow the logical development of the process and be convinced that the results are reasonably 'solid'. The results should be logically presented, plausible, clear, complete without redundancy and should fit with other research. Most importantly, the findings must have 'grab' (Glaser, 1978). They must 'make sense' to the reader, hold the reader's attention and be useful. More specifically, there are some checks that the reader may use to ensure that the theory was rigorously developed. Was variation accounted for and explained, and not simply ignored or not included in the analysis? The commentary surrounding quotations in the text should be thoughtfully rediscussed and brought to a general level of discussion and not left to 'speak for itself', and the researcher should have cited the major authors in the area, connecting the research solidly with the work of others.

Methodological assessment

The first aspect to assess for methodological evaluation is the researcher's approach to the topic. Did the researcher work inductively or did the researcher deductively construct a conceptual framework to sort the data and proceed to analyse the data deductively? Recall that induction does not mean that the researcher must start each investigation from scratch, but may appropriately focus the data collection and analysis within a topic. In the next section, the study by Applegate and Morse (1995), for example, began by focusing on privacy in the nursing home. The study did not, however, define the **components of privacy as a coding system** for sorting data regarding incidents when a resident's privacy was violated, but simply as a topic for inquiry within a very loose definition. Thus, insights were gained into our understanding of privacy as a concept. (For further details, see Sandelowski, 1993, who provides an interesting discussion of the ways that a theoretical knowledge base may be used in qualitative research, without violating principles of induction.)

Data appropriateness and adequacy is ensured by the methods used to sample or to select the research participants. Data **appropriateness** refers to the process of selecting participants who could best inform the research. Were participants selected according to the developing theoretical needs of the study? If a volunteer, convenience or random sampling procedure was used, the sample size should have been large enough to compensate for the secondary selection of participants. This permits the exclusion of those who were not good informants, from whom data are of a particularly poor quality and from whom nothing was learned (Morse, 1991, p. 136). Data **adequacy**, on the other hand, refers to the amount of data obtained and whether or not saturation occurred. Were the findings confirmed with participants or with a secondary sample?

If a standard and well-documented method was used to conduct the study, and if the researcher did not deviate from the methods delineated by other authors, then a detailed description of the methods should not be necessary. However, if the researcher used innovative and less well-documented methods, then a description of how the research was conducted is essential for the evaluation of the study, and the methods should be presented in a clear manner. Methods of coding should be described, and the level of analysis — descriptive or interpretive — should be identified. A short discussion of any problems encountered in the conduct of the study is helpful for those who also wish to investigate this topic.

Consideration of the research process and the 'use of human subjects' in data collection must be considered. Did the investigator adhere to general ethical standards of practice and was clearance obtained from the institutional review boards, from the institution and from the participants themselves? Was the anonymity of the participants (and possible the institution) protected? Were any untoward effects experienced by the participants from participating in the research?

Ultimately, the assessment of the qualitative article is a careful weighing of the strengths and weaknesses of the article. No article is perfect, and the contribution of the article to science is relative. When evaluating an article, it is important to recognize the difficulties that the researcher has encountered in the process of conducting the research, how the researcher surmounted those barriers and the significance of the results.

Utilizing qualitative results in the clinical setting

Inherent in this decision to implement qualitative findings is the question of 'generalizability' of qualitative results. Qualitative research does not have the same standards of replication that quantitative research has for facilitating the decision to adopt research findings. Rather, the process of implementing qualitative research is a wise weighing of the quality of the research (discussed in the previous section), and the relevance of the research to the adoptive setting or context. Some disagree, arguing that because of the limited sample size and the contextual nature of qualitative research, the findings are not applicable to other settings. But if this were truly the case, there would be no point in conducting qualitative research except to solve an immediate problem, and there would certainly be no point in publishing. However, as discussed previously, qualitative results are generalizable, but in a different way from quantitative research. With qualitative methods it is the **theory** that is generalizable to other settings, not like in quantitative research where the strength or significance of the relationships between variables is paramount. Thus the task of the research — and the reader — is the consideration of the article to determine if the qualitative research has relevance, fit and provides an explanation for a similar problem in that particular setting.

For example Applegate and Morse (1995), using ethnography, explored the concept of privacy in a veterans nursing home in Canada. All of the residents were male. The major findings were that respect of privacy depended on the perception that the residents and staff members had in the relationship. That is privacy was respected if the dyad considered each other as a **friend**. When relationships were more formal — as a **stranger** — they still respected the norms of privacy. All of the violations of privacy occurred when one member of the dyad treated the other **as an object**. Now, it is the readers' responsibility to determine if this theory is applicable to their own setting. When making this decision, the most important feature is to consider the nature of interactions in their setting. Do privacy violations occur when residents and staff are not considering the humanness of the other individual? If so, then the study is applicable. Most importantly, the fact that the original study was conducted in a Canadian institution, with an all-male resident population of a certain socio-economic status and health status, **is not important** in making this decision. It is the theory that will be implemented in the setting.

Phenomenological research, exploring the essence of human experience, ensures 'generalizability' or the transferability of the article in the process of exploring the phenomena itself. Recall that phenomenology, in the process of data collection, seeks experiences beyond the immediate conversations with participants, to include relevant descriptions from poetry, literature, art, films and so forth. Thus, the process of incorporating phenomenological findings is essentially the same as for the ethnographic findings, except that the 'context' is one's own experience and one considers the relevance of the results for one's own practice. For example Baron's (1985) study, 'I can't hear you when I'm listening', is a phenomenological study written by a doctor when he found himself in this paradoxical situation while listening to a talkative patient's chest. At one level, the article reflects our values of listening to the body, rather than the person, during physical examination. But we could also, at another level, reflect on this paradox in other situations; that is the actual situation of the study — listening to a patient's chest — may not be a critical part of the experience. Phenomenology make us more empathetic and provides insights into others' experiences while enriching our own. When we read Smith's (1989/92) story of his child's heart surgery, the glimpses of the child's experiences offered to us increases our understanding of paediatric patients and parents in hospitals.

Thus, the evaluation of qualitative results for utilization in the clinical setting does not involve the ritualistic and structured application of a specific protocol but, rather, thoughtful reflection. However, the rather informal application of qualitative findings does not mean that qualitative research does not change the status quo: qualitative research often has a powerful effect on practice, on policy change and, most importantly, on humanistic practice.

PRINCIPLES

- Completed research should be presented to the scientific community both through presentation and publication, otherwise the effort and expense of conducting research is lost.
- When preparing a research report, presentation or article, first clearly identify what it is you want to say and to whom you want to say it.
- Outline the article or presentation, select quotations and prepare any tables or figures before you begin to write.
- Select the journal that will reach your target audience, and review the journal's guidelines so you can write to fit the journal's style.
- Qualitative researchers describe their findings and use data to support their findings so that the reader shares the participants' experiences.
- Researchers must present quotations in order to maintain clarity while protecting anonymity.

- Effective posters catch the eye, limit methods to essentials and focus on the findings.
- The reader is the judge of generalizability or tranferability of the theory to the practice setting.

REFERENCES

Applegate, M. and Morse, J.M. (1995) Personal privacy and interactional patterns in a nursing home. *Journal of Aging Studies*, **8**, 413–34.

Barinaga, M. (1992) Who controls a researcher's files? *Science*, **256**, 1620–1.

Baron, R.J. (1985) An introduction to medical phenomenology: I can't hear you when I'm listening. *Annals of Internal Medicine*, **103**, 606–11.

Bergum, V. (1989/91) Being a phenomenological researcher, in *Qualitative Nursing Research: A Contemporary Dialogue*, rev. edn, (ed. J.M. Morse), Sage, Newbury Park, CA, pp. 55–71.

Chenitz, C. and Swanson, J. (1986) *From Practice to Grounded Theory*, Addison Wesley, Menlo Park, CA.

Field, P.A. and Morse, J.M. (1985) *Nursing Research: The Application of Qualitative Approaches*, Croom Helm, London, UK.

Glaser, B.G. (1978) *Theoretical Sensitivity*, Sociology Press, Mill Valley, CA.

May, K.A. (1989/91) Dialogue: the granting game, in *Qualitative Nursing Research: A Contemporary Dialogue*, rev. edn, (ed. J.M. Morse), Sage, Newbury Park, CA, pp. 240–2.

Minnich, E.K. (1990) *Transforming Knowledge*, Temple University Press, Philadelphia.

Morse, J.M. (1991) Strategies for sampling, in *Qualitative Nursing Research: A Contempory Dialogue*, (ed. J.M. Morse), Sage, Newbury Park, CA, pp. 127–46.

Morse, J.M. and Carter, B. (1995) Enduring to live, enduring to survive: the suffering of a resilient burn survivor. *Holistic Nursing Practice*, 5.

Morse, J.M. and Johnson, J. (1991) *The Illness Experience: Dimensions of Suffering*, Sage, Newbury Park, CA.

Rodgers, B.L. and Cowles, K.V. (1993) The qualitative research audit trail: a complex collection of documentation. *Research in Nursing and Health*, **16**, 219–26.

Sandelowski, M. (1993) Theory unmasked: the uses and guises of theory in qualitative research. *Research in Nursing and Health*, **16**, 1–18.

Smith, S.J. (1989/92) Operating on a child's heart: a pedagogical view of hospitalization, in *Qualitative Health Research*, (ed. J.M. Morse), Sage, Newbury Park, CA, pp. 104–22.

Spradley, J.P. and McCurdy, D.W. (1972) *The Cultural Experience*, Kingsport Press, Kingsport, TN.

Strauss, A. (1978) *Qualitative Analysis for Social Scientists*, Cambridge University Press, Cambridge, MA.

Strauss, A. and Corbin, J. (1990) *Basics of Qualitative Research*, Sage, Newbury Park, CA.

van Manen, M. (1990) *Researching Lived Experience: Human Science for an Action Sensitive Pedagogy*, Althouse, London, Ontario.

FURTHER READING

Ely, M., Anzul, M., Friedman, T. *et al.* (1991) *Doing Qualitative Research: Circles Within Circles*, The Falmer Press, New York.

Knafl, K.A. and Howard, M.J. (1984) Interpreting and reporting qualitative research. *Research in Nursing and in Health*, **7**, 17–24.

Lofland, J. (1974) Styles of reporting in qualitative field research. *The American Sociologist*, **9**, 101–11.

Morse, J.M. (1994) Disseminating qualitative research, in *Disseminating Primary Care Research*, (ed. E. Dunn), Sage, Newbury Park, CA, pp. 59–75.

Morse, J.M. (1993) The perfect manuscript. *Qualitative Health Research*, **3**, 3–5.

Richardson, L. (1990) *Writing Strategies: Reaching Diverse Audiences*, Sage, Newbury Park, CA.

Smedley, C. and Allen, M. (1993) *Getting Your Book Published*, Sage, Newbury Park, CA.

van Manen, M. (1984) Practicing phenomenological writing. *Phenomenology + Pedagogy*, **1**, 36–69.

Williams, A. (1990) Reflections on the making of an ethnographic text. *Studies in Sexual Politics*, No. 29, The University of Manchester, Manchester, UK.

Wolcott, H.F. (1990) *Writing up Qualitative Research*, Sage, Newbury Park, CA.

Appendix A
The qualitative proposal

Janice M. Morse

This proposal was submitted to the National Center for Nursing Research, National Institutes of Health (USA), and funded as a three-year foreign award in 1989 (5 R01 NR02130-03). Proposals are always tailored to the requirements of the targeted granting agency. In this example the proposal was submitted on forms provided by the agency, and therefore the front pages, describing the institution, resources, personnel and budget, have been omitted.

This qualitative proposal is an example of writing that builds a case for the importance of the research topic and for the fact that so little is known about comfort (and the confusion about allied concepts, such as caring). As such, the concept is not mature, thus lending itself to qualitative analysis. In the proposal, Morse makes an argument for the triangulation for three qualitative methods and describes each method and the differences between each method. Although sample size is suggested in the proposal (and this enables budget calculations), it is written that the sample size is only an estimate. Plans for data analysis are described with fictitious examples, so that reviewers, unfamiliar with qualitative analysis, may comprehend the process. Note that, as the number of pages that could be submitted were restricted, Morse has saved space by using a number format for the references, and this serves as an additional function of presenting the text for the reader without interruption. Following the proposal is a copy of the 'pink sheet' — the review panel's evaluation of the proposal.

Defining comfort for the improvement of nursing care

ABSTRACT

What is comfort? For the purposes of this proposal, comfort is defined as two states: a temporal state of well-being and a long-term, more constant state of optimal health. The provision of comfort consists of two components: **caring**, a component that motivates the nurse to initiate the nursing process and provides the humanistic quality of care during procedures; and **nursing tasks** or procedures.

This proposal is for the first phase of a three-stage research programme to investigate comfort. Phase I consists of exploratory and descriptive studies to delineate the construct of comfort and comprises three complementary and interrelated studies. The first two studies examine the individual patient. These consist of a phenomenological study examining the meaning of comfort for patients in various care areas and an ethnoscientific study to elicit the components of comfort. The third study will examine the process of comforting in the work setting, using the methods of grounded theory.

These studies will lay an essential foundation for continuing and future research in Phases II and III of this research programme. Phase II will comprise studies that examine the meaning and methods of comforting in the four domains of nursing (i.e. in human responses to illness, to institutionalization, to therapeutic interventions and to the attainment of health), and Phase III will consist of testing these interventions.

The significance of this work is that the theoretical shift from **nurse caring** to **patient comfort** changes the focus of the research from the nurse to the client. Thus, developing knowledge will be clinically relevant and applicable. In addition, the outcome variable, patient comfort, will be both physiologically and psychologically operationizable and measurable.

A. SPECIFIC AIMS

This application is for funding to conduct a series of studies on comfort, to further delineate the meaning of comfort to the individual and to explicate the process and application of comfort for nursing. Three interrelated studies to examine the meaning, domain and process of comforting, and to explore the relationship of comfort with the construct of caring are proposed. These studies include: (1) a phenomenological study to explore the meaning of comfort to hospitalized patients, (2) a study using ethnoscience to delineate the components of comfort and (3) a grounded theory study to explore the process of providing comfort when the nurse is caring for several patients.

Following the completion of these three studies, further application for funding will be made to The National Center for Nursing Research. Phase II will consist of studies that examine the methods and application of comfort in four main areas of nursing. These areas have been identified as human responses to illness, to institutionalization, to therapeutic interventions and to the attainment of health. Phase III of this research programme will be to develop and test nursing procedures that promote comfort. The ultimate, long-term goal of the research programme is to develop a clinically applicable theory of comfort for nursing.

B. BACKGROUND AND SIGNIFICANCE

The ultimate purpose of nursing practice is to promote comfort for the client. The role of the nurse includes actions ranging from **providing** comfort measures for the patient to those that **support** the patient's own attempts. Comfort is defined as a **state of well-being** that may occur during any stage of the illness–health continuum. At this time, two comfort states have been identified: a temporal state (as in the temporary relief of pain) and a more constant, long-term state that is achieved, for example with the attainment of optimal health. (The insights of Dr G. Ewing and B. Lorencz on this subject are acknowledged. These definitions will be refined as these studies are completed and understanding of the construct of comfort attained.)

This focus on comfort does not contradict the nurse-theorists who argue that the 'essence' of nursing is **caring**.[1,2,3] Although caring has been defined in many ways in the nursing literature, there is agreement that caring is an affect, a feeling of concern or responsibility for others that motivates nursing action.[3–7] There is less agreement, however, that caring encompasses all nursing **actions**, which are referred to as scientific care[8] or technical symbols of care.[9,10] Dunlop[11] noted the inadequacies of a caring paradigm, as nursing theory increasingly tends to 'ignore the body and its associated physical care'. Nevertheless, the caring affect must be present during the conduct of nursing procedures for the tasks to be therapeutic,[12,13] and there is an interdependent relationship between the caring attitude and the conduct of nursing tasks. Thus, in this proposal, caring will be considered as an essential component of comforting. **Providing comfort** includes: (1) a caring attitude (which serves as a motivator so that the comforting process will be initiated), (2) a caring (or humanistic) component of the nursing process and (3) nursing procedures which alter the patient's state of well-being. For the purposes of this research, the process of **comforting the patient** (rather than caring) is perceived to be the purpose of nursing.[14]

Interestingly, the theoretical shift from **nurse caring** to **patient comfort** changes the focus of research from the nurse to the patient or client. Thus, the developing knowledge will be clinically relevant and applicable. In addition, the outcome variable, patient comfort, is both physiologically and psychologically operationizable and measurable. As work progresses, it is expected that alteration in comfort states will be quantifiable using indices of individual measures, such as relaxation, recovery, adaptation, coping or mastery; and, later, using population indices such as morbidity, mortality and health care costs. Therefore, this perspective will have significant implications for the development of an applied nursing theory.

There have been two criticisms about the construct of comfort. The first is that 'making the patient comfortable' implies a passive role for the patient that discourages self-care actions. Although comforting does include the application of nursing therapies to minimize discomfort (in which the patient may adopt a passive role), in this framework comfort also encompasses therapies in which the patient is an active participant, responsible for decisions and actions in the therapeutic process. The second criticism is that many nursing actions, such as giving an injection or assisting with postoperative exercises, may cause discomfort and therefore are antagonistic to the comforting framework. I maintain that such actions are essential in order to assist the patient to attain a state of optimal comfort. Thus, the domain of comfort includes understanding intermediate states of **discomfort** in the process of attaining comfort when the end goal is the client's well-being. It also includes assisting the client to attain well-being in any state of health or illness including providing comfort to the dying.

Implications for nursing

Despite the comparatively short period that nursing research has been conducted, most nursing research has been deductive, hypothesis-testing research. The concepts and theories that are primarily used in nursing research have been acquired from other disciplines, such as psychology, sociology or anthropology, or from physiology or medicine. Descriptive, qualitative research, using analytical induction, is uncommon and has not been used until relatively recently.

The problem with the traditional approach, using concepts and theories acquired from other disciplines, is that there is not always a good 'fit' between the situation in which the concepts were derived and the situations or conditions in which the concepts are used in nursing. One such example is the use of the concept 'culture shock' to describe the experience of admission to hospital.[15] A more recent example is the growing debate on the concepts of 'coping' versus 'mastery'.[16] Furthermore, the domain of nursing is unique, and (as in the case of 'comfort') there is often not an equivalent concept available in another discipline that may be borrowed and appropriately utilized in nursing.

There is an urgent need for concept development using an inductive approach. As this project is focused on comfort and is at the 'core' of nursing, the contribution will be significant and clinically relevant.

C. PRELIMINARY STUDIES AND PROPOSED RESEARCH

Since 1981, Morse and her colleagues have accomplished considerable work, further delineating the components and meaning of comfort in various situations. These projects have focused either on the concept *per se* or on the perception and components of distress and suffering, analysing the factors and the processes that alleviate discomfort.

How does one comfort? In 1983 this investigator identified the components of comfort as the use of touch, talking and listening, or combinations of these actions.[14] Each of these components has distinct and unique characteristics according to the circumstances and perceived needs of the client. However, in this previous study, only healthy subjects were interviewed. Further research is required to examine the meaning of the construct to ill persons across the life span and with various health care needs. Therefore, the objectives of the three studies described in this proposal are:

- to delineate the construct of comfort;
- to identify the components of comfort; and
- to identify the process of comfort.

The achievement of these objectives will provide a theoretical basis for the second part of the research programme, which will evaluate nursing strategies for the provision of comfort. The first objective will be achieved in Study I, a phenomonological study of comfort in sick patients from various patient-care settings, which will allow the investigators to explore the meaning of comfort to ill patients. The methods of ethnoscience (Study II) will enable the investigator to identify the components of comfort, thereby meeting the second objective. The third objective, identifying the process of comforting, will be met using the methods of grounded theory to explicate the stages and phases of the comforting process as perceived by nurses and the patients in Study III.

As previously stated, Phase II of the research programme consists of projects related to nursing strategies for the provision of comfort. These studies have been categorized into four areas (Table A.1) that are considered by this investigator to constitute the domain of nursing. These areas are:

- human responses to illness;
- human responses to institutionalization;
- human responses to therapeutic interventions; and
- human attainment of health, including human responses to maturation, chronicity and disability.

The projects presented in this proposal, delineating the meaning, components, and process of comforting, will provide insights for the identification and the analysis of nursing strategies for the provision of comfort and the evaluation of nursing comfort measures.

Human responses to illness

Studies conducted by this investigator have focused primarily on the perception of pain[17-20] and on the behaviour of the patient experiencing pain.[21-22] Using the psychometric technique of compared comparisons, studies have shown that pain perception can be quantified and that the pain expectation is transmitted culturally and varies between cultures. Using a cross-cultural study of childbirth,[21] pain expectation was shown to be consistent with culturally appropriate pain behaviours.

Human responses to institutionalization

Research conducted in this area has examined primarily the iatrogenic discomfort associated with institutionalization, particularly in the area of patient falls[26-32] and the use of physical restraints.[33,34] Other studies examine patient response to institutionalization, such as difficult patients[25] and the use of television.[24] One graduate student is examining the experience of discharge from a psychiatric institution.[38] The 'falls' research programme is completed, except for collaboration with the UAH (University of Alberta Hospital) Bioengineering Department to develop means to increase environmental safety (by developing a geriatric bed) and to increase nursing surveillance (by developing a bed alarm and a chair alarm).[35] Furthermore, analysis of the videotapes collected as a part of the patient restraint project[33,34] revealed that patients spend a large part of their day waiting — waiting to get into bed or out of bed, waiting for doctors, meals or bedpans — yet little is known of the effect of waiting. This concept is not considered in nursing theory, and an inductive approach to theory development as used in this programme ensures that the theory produced is clinically applicable and relevant.

Human responses to therapeutic interventions

Two graduate students are presently conducting projects in this category, examining patients' responses to an illness event or to medical treatments.[36,37] The fourth project, an extensive cross-cultural project examining traditional healing,[40-43] provided insights into the effect of the comforter as a part of the treatment process (i.e. the placebo effect). Most importantly, it exemplified the importance of religion as a component of the healing process, and investigation should continue in this area.

Table A.1 The application of comfort in four domains of nursing: completed and ongoing research

Human responses to illness:

The perception of painful events[17, 18]
The perception of parturition pain[19-21]
Behavioural indices of postoperative pain in the neonate[22]
The meaning of incontinence[23]

Human responses to institutionalization:

The use of TV in a nursing home[24]
Difficult patients[25]
Patient falls[26-32]
The effect of removing restraints[33-34]
Development of a bed alarm and a geriatric bed[35]

Human responses to therapeutic interventions:

Recovery process following hysterectomy[36]
The experience of a myocardial infarction[37]
The meaning of discharge to psychiatric patients[38]
Traditional Cree medicine for psoriasis[41-43]

Human attainment of health:

Meaning of health in an inner-city community[44]
Adolescents' perception of health[45]
Effect of breast- and bottle-feeding on the Fijian and Fiji Indian neonate[46, 47]
Cultural variation in health care beliefs and values[48, 53]
Transcultural relocation and the refugee experience[54-56]

Human responses to maturational changes, chronicity and disability:

Adolescent response to menarche[57-59]
   development of an attitudinal scale (in process)[60]
Childbirth in Fiji[21]
Breast-feeding: cultural values and beliefs[47, 61-63]
Patterns of feeding[64-66] and weaning[67-69]
Postpartal withholding of colostrum: cross-cultural comparison[70]
Waking behaviours of the normal newborn[71]
Breast-feeding: coping with work (in process)[72, 73]
Breast-feeding in the Alberta Woodland Cree: tradition and change[74]
Interracial variation in growth and development[75, 76]

Human attainment of health

The meaning of health and strategies used to attain or maintain health by the elderly, by adolescents, the poor and various cultural groups have been examined.[45,46] The importance of cultural values and beliefs[47-54] for impeding or facilitating health care and the discrepancies between the health care agenda of the health professionals and the client have been examined. Differences in growth and development for various racial groups and the controversy of genetic and ecological factors that contribute to these differences have been critiqued,[75,76] and the importance for nurses identifying the normal from the abnormal has been examined.

Within this domain, a great deal has been accomplished in the subcategory of **maturational changes**. The stresses of adolescents coping with menstruation in school, the mixed messages of shame and pride received during this time and the inadequate preparation of young adolescents have resulted in several publications.[57-59] This includes an information manual for girls aged 12 to 15 years,[59] intended to ease the psychological distress that girls feel at this time. By making girls more comfortable with this maturational change, it was hoped they might cope better. The construction of a Likert scale is in process,[60] and a survey of normative attitudes, so that the relationship between comfort and coping may be explored further. The cultural values inherent in childbirth[21] and infant feeding have been examined.[61-72] Using anthropological techniques, observing and interviewing mothers, patterns of mixed feeding have been identified.[65,66] Methods for maintaining both lactation and work[72,73] and for understanding the cultural pressures for weaning[68,69] are expected to have an important effect on extending the duration of breast-feeding and improving infant health.

This investigator has not yet conducted research on the maintenance of health in the chronically ill or the disabled patient. Note that these two populations are included within the category 'health'. It is the belief of this investigator that while an individual may have a chronic condition, such as diabetes or asthma, or may be disabled, these patients may still attain a state of optimal health within the limits of their disease or disability. Thus, in this research programme, 'health' is not considered as the 'absence of disease or infirmity' but as a relative state.

Evaluation of research programme

Many of the studies conducted to date have examined the **meaning** or the **experience** of the individual and, therefore, primarily qualitative methodologies have been utilized. Because understanding of a phenomenon is derived from intensive interviewing, listening and analysing transcripts, or from observational research, all projects listed are those for which the applicant has served as principal investigator, co-investigator, or supervisor and can access the raw data. As the ultimate goal of this research programme is the inductive development of nursing theory, it is essential that the approach to this initial phase be exceedingly broad, exploratory and descriptive. At present, 'meta-analysis' of multiple qualitative studies conducted in various settings, which investigate differing nursing and patient problems, reveals some common characteristics associated with the experience of illness. This work will be facilitated by further delineating comfort, by linking this knowledge with the experience of patients and carers, by testing this knowledge quantitatively and by applying this information in the practice setting. By using these strategies, nursing practice will advance.

At the moment, there are major weaknesses and gaps in this research programme. There needs to be further research to explicate the construct of comfort. The proposed phenomenological study (Study I below) investigating the meaning of comfort in patients with various types of illnesses must be completed before further analysis of the human responses is continued. Furthermore, as the components of comfort have only been explored in a healthy sample, this study needs to be replicated with a sample of hospitalized patients (Study II). A third study will investigate the process of comforting, using grounded theory. Finally, funding has been obtained from another source for a project entitled, 'Gift-giving in the patient–nurse relationship: reciprocity for care?' The theoretical context of this study suggests that as nurses work for the hospital (and are reimbursed by the hospital), they are perceived to **give** care to patients. Inhibiting the patients' opportunity to reciprocate this care may foster patient dependency on the nurse and contribute to nurse burn-out. Thus, it is important to understand the context of the nurse–patient relationship, yet this aspect is virtually unexplored. These three studies, combined, should delineate comfort as a construct and provide a strong theoretical basis for theory development.

D. STUDY DESIGNS AND METHODS

Study I The meaning of comfort

Presently, there is disagreement about caring theory, including the action or procedural component of nursing. Some authors argue that caring is only an affective response of the nurse,[4,77] while others consider caring to include all behaviours inherent in the nursing process, including the procedural tasks.[6] However, as it is possible for nurses to continue to nurse and to 'do their job' without caring[12] (although such procedures may not be considered 'therapeutic'), caring alone is an inadequate concept to describe nursing behaviours. In this proposal, the first definition of caring will be used: that is, caring will be considered an affect or emotive response of the nurse that compels action;[4] the motivator for nursing action and the humanistic component of care. Caring remains throughout the nursing procedure, but the label for the total action, for caring plus the nursing procedure, is comfort.

Recognizing the importance of the nurse's need to provide comfort for patients, the National Center for Nursing Research funded a conference entitled, 'Key aspects of comfort: management of pain, fatigue and nausea', on 24–26 March, 1988. The majority of the papers presented pertained to the measurement, assessment or the nursing management of pain, fatigue and nausea. A few presenters described patients' self-comforting measures (e.g. 'Burn patients' behaviours to manage pain' [Vanden Bosch]), and although one researcher described the nurses' role in **comforting** ('Comforting the child in pain' [Hester]), only two investigators examined a broader perspective of comfort ('Effects of home nursing care on patients' symptoms and functional status' [McCorkle, Benoliel, Donaldson and Goodell] and 'Perceptions of comfort by the chronically ill hospitalized elderly' [Hamilton]).[78]

This conference signifies a milestone for nursing. Hamilton's[78] presentation made important practical recommendations for change in her comfort themes relating to the disease process, self-esteem, positioning, staff approaches, hospital routine and the lack of privacy, but, as others have done,[79] she did not attempt to develop a definition of comfort. Therefore, this and other applied research may be premature if we are unsure what comfort **is** and what the comfort goal of a nursing intervention **is**.

Presently, comfort is included in many of the nurse-theorists' models of caring. For example comfort is the first of Leininger's major taxonomic caring constructs,[80,p.138] but again, comfort is not defined. Watson *et al.*[81,p.39] associate comfort with 'safety and security'; Ray writes of comfort as a physical characteristic[9,p.108] and equates caring with comfort for the relief of pain.[10] 'To make my relative comfortable' was included in Mayer's[82] list of cancer patients' perceptions of nurse-caring behaviours. In a national survey on the caring content of baccalaureate curricula, Selvin and Harter[77] noted that comfort was included in 81.8% of the programmes surveyed and was exceeded only by support (86.7%), stress alleviation (87.5%), trust (89.4%) and coping (93.2%). Therefore, given the recognized importance of comfort, the lack of a definition and the lack of research in this area is a serious concern.

This study will elicit the human experience of comforting, of being comforted and of being made comfortable. What is comfort? And what does it mean to feel (or to be) comfortable? How does one **know** when one is comfortable? How long does a comfort state last before discomfort returns? What are self-comforting measures? Can comfort be achieved by oneself? Is it a state of mind, a physiological state or both?

Method

Phenomenology is the method of choice when seeking to **understand, make sense** and elicit the meaning of a phenomenon,[83] and it is described by Husserl as the study of the meaning of human experience. Ray[84] summarizes the main characteristics of the phenomenological method as: (1) focusing on the nature of the lived experience; (2) holding in abeyance one's scientific presuppositions about a phenomenon; (3) conducting intense dialogues with people about the meaning of an experience; (4) developing themes from recorded dialogues; and (5) reflecting deeply on the meaning of the whole experience.

Subject selection

A purposeful sample of approximately 10 hospitalized participants will be selected according to: (1) their ability to participate (i.e. their willingness and desire to commit time to be interviewed, their ability to express themselves and their willingness to share their experiences with the researcher); and (2) their experience with comfort and discomfort in relation to their disease/illness state. For example the researcher will seek one geriatric stroke patient, one patient with a myocardial infarction, one orthopaedic patient in traction (bed-bound), one patient with a terminal illness, one post-surgical patient with a major chest or abdominal incision, one patient in the burn unit, one patient with chronic respiratory problems and one patient with multiple trauma. The purpose is to seek out informants with divergent experiences of physical comfort and discomfort, so that a comprehensive description of comfort may be obtained. Although (based on a study by Bergum)[85] it is anticipated that 10 informants will be adequate to obtain comprehensive descriptions, additional informants may be added until the investigator is satisfied that the data are complete.

Data collection

At the beginning of each interview, an explanation of the study will be given and consent to participate in the study will be obtained (Appendix A, Consent Form). The participants will be informed that they are not required to participate in the study, that they may stop the interview at any time or refuse to answer any questions, and that whether or not they participate will have no bearing on the care they receive. The participants will be assured of anonymity, and, although some of the information they provide will be published, their names will not be associated with the publication.

Next, demographic data will be obtained from each patient. Information on the patient's age, sex, level of education, marital status, number of children and occupation will be obtained. From the patient's chart, the past and current medical history will be obtained and, from the nursing care plan, a listing of nursing measures ordered. This information will be used to describe the sample and to ensure the informant has had experiences that will enrich the data.

Multiple tape-recorded, open-ended, interactive interviews will be conducted with each participant. Whenever possible, these interviews will be conducted in the 'quiet room' of a unit so that the participant will be assured of privacy without interruption. At the beginning of the interview, the informants will be asked broad questions and encouraged to respond in narrative form. For example opening questions may be: 'Tell me about your illness from the beginning ...'. Such a strategy of encouraging in-depth descriptions of the illness experience **in total** prevents the researcher from prematurely narrowing the informant's definition of comfort. Gentle probes will be asked in order to enrich the description of the experience and to focus the interview.

An example of this interviewing process (using fictitious data and a situation adapted from Lear)[86,p.336] is:

> Informant: I walked out of the unit. A woman came and embraced me. She felt plump and warm. She led me back to the waiting room, her hand holding mine, and talking steadily and soothingly. She said her name was Bonnie. She was the head nurse. It was not yet hopeless. Quite true, it was very bad, but it was not yet hopeless. They had done this and that, and such and so had happened, he had not responded, but they were going to continue trying, and I was to wait in the waiting room and not lose hope, not lose hope, and she would come back and tell me, she said, whatever more there was to tell, as soon as there was anything more to tell. And in this way she sat me down, and petted me, and plumped herself about me, as though she were a comforter. I wanted to sink into her and sleep.
> Researcher: (asking a probe) And you felt ...?
> Informant: EXHAUSTED! I was **so** exhausted I couldn't focus, I couldn't think, I couldn't feel! There was a buzz in my head — I couldn't comprehend, couldn't believe what was happening, that it was actually happening. But I trusted Bonnie, I knew she would keep me on keel, that she would make sure I knew of any changes, that everything was being done as she said, and she would steer me through this, I just had to do as she said. So I waited, trying to make sense, trying to accept.

The initial description of the illness experience is expected to take one or two hours. After this has been obtained, the researcher will begin the analysis, returning to re-interview the participant about specific comfort themes as they emerge from the data.

It may be possible that some of the data may be obtained by investigating the converse of comfort (i.e. by examining **discomfort**). For instance if one of the participants focuses on **waiting** (such as waiting for a bedpan, waiting for dinner, waiting for the doctor, waiting for visitors, waiting for an analgesic, waiting-all-night-for-the-morning and so forth), then the researcher will return to other participants for information on this concept and to verify agreement or disagreement about this theme. 'Comfort', then, in relation to this theme would be 'managing waiting'. Thus, insights will be added by understanding what comfort is **not**.

Data analysis

Intra-participant analysis

In phenomenology, the first step in data analysis is immersion in the data **as a whole**. This is achieved by listening to the tapes and by extensive reading and rereading of the transcripts. The researcher then **reflects on these data in their entirety.**[87] The meaning of each sentence is considered in the light of the complete transcript, and statements that appear particularly revealing will be highlighted (van Manen).[88] Thus, a disciplined and systematic search is performed for descriptive expressions that are identified as 'at the centre' of the experience.[89] These experiences, themes or constituents,[85] are continually rephrased, their relevance confirmed, and then they are described in a few sentences. (Note that this interpretative process differs from the content analysis used in ethnography or grounded theory, where significant similar portions of data are removed and combined in a separate file.) For instance the comforting behaviour offered by the nurses may be interpreted as 'removing responsibility'. In the above example (adapted from Lear),[86] the nurse, guided by physically supporting and touching, was honest about the patient's condition yet suggested hope 'not be lost', kept communication open by keeping the relative informed, did not isolate the relative and suggested appropriate behaviours ('Wait here.') when the informant was incapable of making decisions herself. The outcome was a feeling of relaxation, fatigue and a desire to sleep. Note that a significant aspect of phenomenological research is maintaining the experience in totality. The comforting strategies are not separated but rather kept in context. The researcher interprets and confirms each participant's experience before seeking inter-participant commonalties.

Inter-participant analysis

In the next stage of analysis, the researcher seeks for commonalties between participants, gathering statements that are conceptually similar,[89] and it is these inter-participant themes that constitute the 'essence' of the phenomena or meta-theme. Although some of the themes will be common to all participants, some of the themes will not (i.e. there will be unique themes). It is these unique themes that provide the variation and enrich the data with the range of experiences that are manifest in various disease/illness states. For this reason, a heterogeneous sample of patients with various nursing needs were selected.

Interrelationships between themes

The third phase of data analysis is to seek interrelationships between the meta-themes and descriptions, using quotes from the interviews as concrete illustrations to provide a realistic and accurate portrayal of the phenomena for the reader. The process of writing and rewriting increases the insights and the reflections of the reader, facilitating interpretation. To ensure validity, the analysis will then be given back to the participants for verification, and any areas of disagreement, of inadequate description or omissions will be further interpreted and corrected.

Ray[90] summarizes this process of phenomenological reductionism as a reflective, analytical process of identification (i.e. uncovering the constituents of the experience), intentionality (i.e. the essential character of 'property of acts' directed towards the object), discounting or bracketing (i.e. delimiting the experience and removing preconceptions and a priori knowledge) and intuition (i.e. insight). This process of structured reflection takes place between the nurse (ego) and the 'concrete inquiry of the universe of nursing'.

Tesch[89] stresses that the process of phenomenological research is one of questioning, and one that requires substantial 'reflection, readiness, openness and immersion' on the part of the investigator. A theme is valid and complete only when there is a deep feeling of satisfaction that the results are right and the ideas solid. Ray[90] notes that validity is 'formulated in the light of the client's conceptions of him or herself in the world', and are valid 'if recognised as true by those who live the experience'. Thus, because of the reflexive nature of the phenomenological process, that phenomenological inquiry cannot be 'forced'. Although this study will commence first, in order to allow enough time for this process of reflection and interpretation to occur, the study will extend over the total project period of three years.

Study II The components of comfort

This study will be a replication and extension of the 1983 study[14] that examined the components of comfort in four healthy women, aged between 23 and 29 years. The pilot study explored the parameters and the dimensions of comfort and determined the feasibility of using ethnoscience, a linguistic technique, to examine a non-verbal behaviour, such as comfort.

In the pilot study, the domain of comfort was shown to have two main segregates, **touching** and **talking**, and a minor segregate, **listening**. Each of these segregates was used for particular situations. **Touching** was used alone if the person was perceived to be feeling unloved or afraid; **touching with a little talking**, was used if the person was sick or in pain; **talking with a little touching** was used if the person felt insecure, afraid or depressed; **talking** (without touching) was used if the person was lonely, bored, rejected or lacked confidence, and **listening** was used if the person was frustrated or angry. Each of the methods of comforting was used according to the relationship between the comforter and the person in need of comfort and the seriousness of the situation. For example it was considered appropriate for a wife to comfort her husband using touch (especially in a private situation), but inappropriate for a stranger to provide comfort using touch, unless in extremely stressful situations, such as the scene of a car accident. Comfort may be offered more freely to children, anywhere. In this study some information was obtained on self-comforting strategies, primarily praying and talking to oneself for reassurance or using distraction. The outcome of comforting was described as a change in mood, as a 'warm feeling of relief', 'feeling confident', 'in touch with self' and 'at ease.'[14]

This pilot study showed that although comfort was a non-verbal behaviour, phrases could be used to describe actions for which the English language does not have descriptors (e.g. types of comforting, such as 'touching with a little talking') and that meaningful information could be obtained using ethnoscience. However, the main limitation of this study was that it was conducted with healthy young females, and these data pertained mostly to a normal, healthy, everyday life. Do patients who are ill or in chronic or acute pain, dependent on nursing for assistance with personal body functions, perceive comfort in the same way? Does the elderly patient or the male patient have a different perspective on comfort? It is clear that additional research must be conducted on the components of comfort before additional work continues.

Method

Ethnoscience is the method of choice when the aim of the study is to elicit the characteristics of a domain. Ethnoscience consists of linguistic techniques for identifying from interview data, the characteristics and the types of 'things' by contrasting and distinguishing features 'that are real, significant, meaningful, accurate, or in some other fashion regarded as appropriate by the actors themselves'.[91] The major assumption in the method is that informants 'make sense of their world' using formal patterning of behaviours and models that are consistent and shared through culture. These patterns may be elicited through unstructured, interactive interviews and by analytical linguistic techniques, such as comparative questioning and card sorts.[92-94]

Sample selection

A purposeful or theoretical sample of 10 young adult patients from each of the medical and surgical areas and 10 patients from the long-term care units, including 10 geriatric patients (i.e. ~40) will serve as primary informants. These informants will be selected by the investigator according to their ability to articulate and their willingness to participate in the study. Interviews will be conducted in the areas of the patient's choice, either at the bedside or in the unit 'quiet room'. Following the methods of purposeful sampling, additional informants will be selected according to the theoretical needs of the research as data analysis progresses. Emphasis will be on the depth of knowledge and experience within informants, rather than eliciting superficial information for a large number of subjects.

Following standard procedure, at the beginning of each interview an explanation of the study will be given and consent to participate in the study will be obtained (Appendix A). The participants will be informed that they are not required to participate in the study, that they may stop the interview at any time or refuse to answer any questions, and that whether or not they participate will have no bearing on the care they receive. The participants will be assured of anonymity, and, although some of the information they provide will be published, their name will not be associated with the publication.

In order to describe the sample, demographic data will also be obtained from each patient (Appendix C). This information will consist of the patient's age, sex, level of education, marital status, number of children and occupation. From the patient's chart, past and current medical history will be obtained and, from the nursing care plans, a listing of nursing measures ordered that provide comfort.

Procedure

The ethnoscience method involves multiple interviews with each informant, and data analysis is ongoing throughout data collection. Because of the process nature of data collection and analysis, these procedures will be described together as an ongoing and interactive process.[83,94–96]

In the first interview session, the domain (or boundaries of the category) is identified by asking informants such questions as: 'Tell me about a time when you felt comfortable', 'How do you know when you are comfortable?', 'When were you last uncomfortable?', 'Is feeling discomfort different from feeling uncomfortable?' and 'What makes **you** feel comfortable?'

When using this method, because the investigator is **learning and exploring the domain with the informant**, the interview and the examples used are not the same for each informant. Rather, the investigator analyses the information from the first informant and progresses using these descriptions with the next informant, occasionally confirming or expanding any areas considered 'thin'. The assumption is that because the information is culturally shared (although not necessarily previously overtly expressed) the information may be elicited from any informant. Thus, the investigator is actually beginning to analyse these data **during the interview**. As information is learned, the investigator places the information within the context of what is already known, examines it and plans subsequent questions. When two or more areas for exploration are realized, these questions are retained. An expert interviewer can follow one line of investigation and, when that area is complete, return and pursue the second line of investigation. As such, this form of inquiry requires intense concentration and is exhausting for both the interviewee and the investigator. Not more than two interviews should be conducted on any one day. Fatigue seriously decreases the quality of the interview and the information obtained.

When presented to a member of the group, valid information is instantly recognized as 'correct' and may be confirmed and expanded upon by eliciting different perspectives or examples according to the informant's experiences.

Interviews are tape recorded, and the principal investigator will be available for listening to the interviews and advising the research assistants. Regular meetings will be conducted with the assistants to ensure the use of rigourous interviewing techniques. Interviews will be immediately transcribed, and data will be entered into a microcomputer.

Card sorts

The first formal analysis is to identify descriptors that appear in the data, and the investigator creates lists of these words. For example one list may be descriptors on types of patients, another on the kinds of nursing approaches and so forth. When the first round of interviews has been completed, these lists are transferred to cards (in triplicate) for the card-sort procedures that are conducted during the second interviews. This is the first step in developing a taxonomy.

At the beginning of the second round of interviews, again the interviewer may commence using open-ended questions to obtain further information to expand upon the first interview. Then, the informant is given one set of the prepared cards to sort into as many piles as the informant chooses. The tape recorder is left on and the informant is asked to think out loud as the task is performed. When completed, the interviewer questions the informant about the sorting order: 'Why did you put these cards together?', 'What do these cards have in common?', 'What is the difference between this pile and this pile?' and 'Please name this pile'. Elastic bands are placed around the cards, so that the sort is retained for later recording.

During the second round, the informant is asked to do a **triadic card sort**, this time sorting the cards into three piles. Again the sort procedure is tape recorded so that information may be obtained about the similarities and differences between the piles, and the stacks are labelled and saved for analysis. Finally, in the **dyadic card sort**, the cards are forced into two piles and the interview procedure is repeated.

Development of a taxonomy

The card sort procedure enables the identification of segregates (i.e. similar items or categories) and subsegregates, which form levels of the taxonomy. For example under the domain of 'types of comfort', the investigator should be able to identify several main groups and the subsegregates that fit under each type. Analysis of the tape-recording will provide the characteristics of each type, and the conditions (for whom, where and why) for which each nursing measure is used.

The purpose of the third interview is to obtain further information on any areas that are still shallow or skimpy, and to share the taxonomy with the informant for verification. Again the interview is tape recorded and transcribed. The informant is carefully questioned about the taxonomy, and any areas of agreement noted and concerns or disagreement carefully documented.

If the latter occurs, and the informant has reservations about the taxonomy, the research continues with additional informants being sought until the model is validated.

Content analysis

This is also performed on the interview data after each interview, in order to fully describe the context of the study. Data will be uploaded from floppy discs to the mainframe for the use of $QUAL,$[92] a program that facilitates content analysis after coding.* First-level codes, or descriptors of important components of the interviews, are noted in the margins. Then, using the smallest number of categories, data will be coded and the portions of transcripts for these codes extracted. If each category provides a substantial amount of information, the category may then be recoded. For example if a category, such as 'non urgent patient needs', is large, it may be further subdivided into smaller categories, such as 'things patients should be encouraged to do themselves' and 'things that nurses are expected to do for patients'. Of course, as the data are not yet collected at this point, these category names are hypothetical.

The final stage of the analysis is the identification of **specific statements**, **general statements** and **abstract statements**. Specific statements are propositions derived from those data that appear to be correct, and may be subjected to further testing as hypotheses in subsequent research. Following the second round of interviews, group meetings will be held to compare data from various areas, to develop hypotheses, to elicit differences and to identify commonalities between patient care areas. General statements may also be subsequently tested or verified during the third round of interviews. They are broader than specific statements and may also be used as research questions in a future study. Abstract statements are the highest level, and should form the initial steps in theory development or contribute to existing theory.

---

* $QUAL$[92] computer techniques have removed the mechanical tasks of cutting, pasting and sorting from qualitative analysis. However, present programs available for microcomputers, while ideal for small studies, are still inadequate for large projects. File sizes are limited (especially if a hard disk drive is unavailable) and typical printing facilities are often too slow for convenient proofing of data and receiving results. Researchers have found innovative, but less than ideal, ways to overcome these problems, such as splitting the text data into multiple smaller files (but this is awkward in practice) or abstracting data for analysis.[95] If more data than could be transcribed or handled is collected, some authors have even randomly selected the interviews to be included in the analysis (Prescott, Dennis and Jacox).[96] $QUAL$ was written for a mainframe computer to permit the handling of large data sets to overcome the limitations of microcomputer packages. When using $QUAL$, data are easy to code and may be retrieved by interview, subject, question or code(s), and the investigator has the option of designating retrieval order. In running the program three files are specified: a question file, a database file containing the transcribed interviews and an output file containing the results of a search.

Study III Explication of the process of comforting

Significant advances in nursing over the past decades have changed nursing from a technical, procedure-based apprenticeship to a profession focused on therapeutic interventions. Although the purpose of these interventions is to enhance patient comfort, little is known about this process.

The only work in this area was conducted by Strauss and his colleagues,[97,p.153] who noted the paradoxical situation where nursing comfort tasks are routinely scheduled and conflict with medical interventions which inflict **discomfort**. Because of the acute care and curing orientation of the hospital, nursing comfort tasks are devalued and regarded by the patients as non-technical, ordinary, kind and helpful.[p.156] Thus comfort work becomes invisible despite its therapeutic implications, and when nurses are overworked, comfort work receives lower priority in the work schedule than medical/technical tasks.

Strauss *et al.* identified five types of comfort work tasks for nursing: (1) preparing the patients for discomfort, (2) assessing discomfort, (3) preventing discomfort, (4) minimizing discomfort and (5) relieving discomfort.[p.157] Comfort tasks for patients include: (1) legitimating discomfort (2) enduring discomfort and (3) expressing discomfort.[97,p.157]

A recent study conducted by Estabrook[98] examined the use of touch in intensive care, using grounded theory. The core variable identified in this study was **cueing**, i.e. 'a process by which ... one determines the need for, the appropriateness of, anticipates the response to, and evaluates the effects of touch.'[p.100] Negative cues from the patient cause the nurse to withdraw touch, while positive cues are indicative that the touch is meeting a need and should continue. Do nurses use a process similar to cueing to determine which is the most comforting or comfortable approach? What is the process of comforting?

Method

For this study, the methods of grounded theory[99-103] will be employed, using interactive unstructured interviews and participant observation. This is the method of choice when the construct being examined is considered a dynamic process.

Sample selection

As the styles of comforting may differ by age of the patient and patient care area, purposeful sampling will be used. Three samples of informants will be used for this study.

- Approximately five nurses will be selected from each of five patient care areas — paediatrics, adult medical, adult surgical and geriatrics and palliative care (n ~ 25). Because this study will not commence until June 1990, the units that will be involved in this study will be negotiated closer to the starting date.

- Patients who are also nurses will be selected (n ~ 10). Although there are reports of physicians' care by physicians who are patients,[104] reports from nurses evaluating their colleagues' care are absent in the literature. Nurses who are patients have been deliberately selected for the study, for, as nurses, they know what should be done under ideal conditions, what they received and did not receive while a patient. They will, therefore, be in an ideal position to evaluate both sides of the issue and will make excellent informants.

- Nurses who are also relatives of patients will be selected (n ~ 10). As a relative, the informant is not in the vulnerable position of the patient, and relatives frequently serve as advocates for patients.[105] Relatives have time to be observant and to watch nurses caring for many patients, while patients may focus only on the care they have been provided. In order to identify patients and relatives who are also nurses, a request for study participants will be placed in *NUVO* (*Nurses' Voice*), an internal monthly newsletter distributed to all hospital staff, requesting the assistance of nursing staff in identifying potential participants. In addition, signs will be posted in the patient lounges and waiting rooms.

Following the methods of purposeful sampling, additional informants will be selected according to the theoretical needs of the research as data analysis progresses. Again, emphasis will be on the depth of knowledge (rather than breadth) and the experience of informants.

Procedure

As for the previous studies, at the beginning of each interview an explanation of the study will be given and consent to participate in the study will be obtained. The participants will be informed that they are not required to participate in the study, that they may stop the interview at any time or refuse to answer any questions. The participants will be assured of anonymity and that, although some of the information they provide will be published, their name will not be associated with the publication.

Next, demographic data will be obtained from each participant. This will consist of age, sex, level and type of education (including nursing education), marital status, number of children and present occupation. From those participants who are patients, the past and current medical history will be obtained from the chart. This information will be used to describe the sample.

Open-ended, interactive interviews will be conducted to determine the nurses', patients' and relatives' perceptions of care. These interviews will be conducted during the nurses' own time, in the quiet room on the unit or in the investigator's office. Multiple tape-recorded interviews will be conducted with each informant, and data analysis will continue throughout data collection.

During the first interview, the topic will be approached broadly by asking informants such questions as, 'Tell me about a typical day'. Next, depending on the data obtained from the first interviews, the interviews will become more focused. For example questions may be: 'Tell me how you would comfort a distressed elderly female patient who is confused, an elderly man in pain, a patient who is irritated from waiting, a patient who rings her bell unnecessarily and constantly, when you need to ask an adolescent to turn the TV down, a depressed patient who has had bad news and a patient who is "fed up" with lying in bed?'

Patients who are also nurses will be asked: 'Tell me what it is like to be in hospital: Is it what you expected? What nursing care measures do you find helpful ... unhelpful? What nursing care approaches relieve your discomfort ... are unhelpful ... make it worse?' Relatives will be asked about their experience as an observer of the comforting process and the experience of being a passive observer of care. To enhance the process of constant comparison, a separate research assistant will conduct the interviews in each of the five patient care areas.

Participant observation will also be conducted in several care areas, both at busy times and slack times. Furthermore, spot observation[83,106] will be conducted on many units to confirm findings as the study progresses. During these periods of observation, the researchers will subjectively record the comforting tasks and perceived responses of patients. The nurses' notion of the importance and the ordering of tasks will be recorded. Field-notes or descriptions of observations will be entered into the laptop microcomputer at regular intervals.

Data analysis

Again, all interviews are transcribed and data analysis conducted by uploading files from the microcomputer and implementing $QUAL^{92}$ to manage this large data set.

The process of data analysis in grounded theory uses the constant comparative method which facilitates the identification of patterns. Incidents are compared with incidents, incident with category, and category with category or construct.[102,p.122] Thus, basic properties of the category are defined, the relationships between the categories identified and the properties and conditions — causes, contexts and consequences — made explicit. Next, the researcher compares this patterning within different groups so that clusters are delineated. Incidents/participants that do not fit within the schema are considered 'negative cases' and purposefully sorted out and interviewed to increase the variability or understanding of the scope of the category. Note that there is an interaction between data collection and data analysis, with each providing the direction for the other. The process of **memoing** enables the documentation of theoretical ideas, insights and interpretations throughout the process of data collection. These index cards, or memos, enhance the process of conceptualization and modification of the theory.

As data are collected, the categories become descriptive, and linkages, or the relationships between the categories, are identified. Descriptions of typical events and patterns of behaviour may be identified and summarized. As the level of interpretation increases, so the theory becomes more abstract. The data are considered 'saturated' when no new data or instances can be identified and the category is 'coherent', or makes sense. The core variable, or the variable that explains most of the process, becomes the basis for the emerging theory. A core variable may be a condition, a consequence or a process. If the process has two or more stages, changes over time, and these changes create discrete demarcation points, this process is termed a 'basic social structural process' (**BSSP**). A psychological process is termed a 'basic social psychological process' (**BSPP**). Thus, if comforting is a process, with stages and phases, the basic social psychological process identified will be inextricably related to the core variable. Diagramming will assist in making the categories, hypothesized linkages and relationships explicit.[99,100]

At this stage, the researcher returns to the library to seek information in the literature, so that links to established theory can be identified. According to Glaser and Strauss,[99] in addition to the other criteria for evaluating theory (i.e. logical consistency, clarity, parsimony, density and scope), the theory should be relevant and able to predict and explain the data under study and fit the situation being researched.

Reliability and validity

One of the most important steps for the maintenance of reliability and validity in qualitative research is the selection of the sample.[107] A purposeful or theoretical sample will be selected according to the experience of the informant (i.e. the amount and type of knowledge the informant has and the theoretical needs of the study) and the qualities of the informant (i.e. the ability and willingness to be interviewed). To ensure that the data will be 'rich', informants from various areas will be selected. Hence, the study will meet the criteria of **adequacy**.[100] The interviewing (and sampling) will continue until these data are saturated or becomes repetitive. Thus, the test for **adequacy** of data will be met.[100] Data will be verified with secondary informants, and negative cases or exceptions will be sought. Thus, the investigator will obtain a sample that will be able to represent the population according to the knowledge domain rather than according to demographic characteristics. Because of this, the results may not be generalizable in the usual sense that the sample may be atypical. However, as the level of interpretation becomes increasingly abstract, the theoretical generalizability increases. Thus, later testing and refining of the results may show that the theoretical findings are applicable in other settings, and thus the study has external validity.[101,p.291]

Issues of internal validity include, first, the problem of interviewer bias. One criticism of qualitative research is that interviewers are able to see 'evidence' of anything they wish to find by asking leading questions. Several techniques assist in the removal of interviewer bias. The first is the concept of 'bracketing', or consciously identifying researchers theoretical biases and placing those aside.[108,109] Lincoln and Guba[110] refer to this as neutrality or objectivity in the manner in which the question is framed. Kvale[109] notes that the lack of standardization in the interviews actually increases validity, for it ensures that the researchers are asking the 'right' questions in a meaningful fashion. If the researcher is not, the informant can ask for clarification. Furthermore, the investigator may later examine the transcripts and analyse any leading questions and the type of responses received. Therefore, the 'solution appears not to work towards technical objectivity, but rather a reflected subjectivity with respect to the question-answer interactions'.[p.190]

A second concern is that the interviewers may not be consistent in their interviewing techniques and may vary in sensitivity. This is also considered advantageous, as it 'gives a broader and more richly nuanced picture of themes to be focused upon'.[109,p.189] A decrease in intersubjectively reproducible information, while reliable in the traditional sense, actually provides richer data and increases validity. However, issues of accuracy are of concern. All interviews will be checked for gaps to identify any areas that have been omitted. Following the transcription, the interviews will be checked by the researcher to ensure that the typist has correctly transcribed the interview and has included notations for all pauses, exclamations, and otherwise indicated as much of the informant's expression as possible.

During data analysis, the problem is to decide whether or not interpretations are acceptable or superficial, simplistic, one-sided or distorted. There is a difference between scoring the reliability of a test and assessing the reliability of interpretation, and, for this reason, it does not assist the qualitative researcher to use multiple coders or to recode to assess reliability. First, variation may occur in the analysis according to whether the investigator considers that the purpose is to determine the interviewee's intended meaning (and use latent content analysis) or to determine what the text has to say to us (and therefore use manifest coding analysis). Second, variation in analysis may occur because there is a legitimate plurality of interpretations (as with the current debate over the interpretation of the New Testament).[109] If plural interpretations are acknowledged as being possible, then it is meaningless to use strict criteria for analysis. Rather, the investigator must leave explicit, detailed evidence between the indicators in the data and the conceptualization of the analytic categories.[111]

Summary of research methods

In the following table, the research methods for each study are summarized:

Table A.2 Comparison of three methods proposed to explore comfort

Procedure	Methods		
	Study I *Phenomenology*	*Study II* *Ethnoscience*	*Study III* *Grounded theory*
Sample	Purposeful	Purposeful	Purposeful
Participants	~ 10 patients from various areas	~ 40 med/surg areas including 10 geriatric	~ 25 nurses ~ 10 patients-who-are-nurses ~ 10 relatives-who-are-nurses
Informed consent	Yes	Yes	Yes
Demographic data	Yes	Yes	Yes
Data collection	Tape recorded, interactive	Interactive interviews Dyadic/triadic sorts	Interactive interviews Participant observation Field-notes, diary
Data analysis	Interviews transcribed Search for themes and inter-relationships between themes	Interviews transcribed Content analysis (QUAL) Prepare taxonomy Develop: • specific statements • general statements • abstract statements Develop theory	Interviews transcribed Constant comparison (*QUAL*) Develop categories Identify: • core variable • linkages between • categories • *BSPP*
Reliability and validity	Verify with participants	Verify using card sorts Seek negative cases	Verify with observation Check with secondary informants Theory: • fit? • work?
Results	Description of meaning of comfort	Description of components of comfort	Description of process of comfort

Timeline

The scheduled programme of work is as follows:

Table A.3 Timeline

Study	Year 1	Year 2	Year 3
Study I			
Hire staff			
Data collection	XXXXXXXXXXXXXXXXXXXXXXXX		
Data analysis	XXXXXXXXXXXXXXXXXXXXXXXX		
Preparation of			
the final report			XXXXXX
Study II			
Hire staff	XX		
Data collection	XXXXXX		
Data analysis	XXXXXX		
Preparation of			
the final report	XXXXX		
Study III			
Hire staff		XX	
Data collection		XXXXXXXXXXX	
Data analysis		XXXXXXXXXXX	
Preparation of			
the final report			XXXXXXX

Researcher

The most critical aspect for considering a qualitative proposal for funding depends upon the ability of the investigators to complete the study successfully, to utilize rigorous methods, to elicit significant data and to build a credible, useful and unique theory.

The principal investigator in this study has conducted previous work on comfort and is involved with the development of qualitative methods in nursing. She has previously co-authored a text on qualitative methods and published two chapters on sampling. In November 1987, she organized a symposium in Chicago that brought the leading qualitative methodologists together for a two day think-tank. This meeting will result in a publication, *Qualitative Methods: A Contemporary Dialogue*, (Aspen). She has taught qualitative methods at the graduate level for six years and, in Studies II and III, she will employ graduate thesis students as research assistants so they may gain experience using qualitative methods.

E. HUMAN SUBJECTS

This research will be conducted with full consideration for the rights of human subjects. Only adults over the age of 18 years will be included in this ⸀research.

Patients

As stated, at the beginning of each interview an explanation of the study will be given and consent to participate in the study will be obtained. The participants will be informed that they are not required to participate in the study, that they may stop the interview at any time or refuse to answer any questions, and that whether or not they participate will have no bearing on the care they receive. The participants will be assured of anonymity, and, although some of the information they provide will be published, their names will not be associated with the publication. They will be given a copy of the informed consent form (see Appendix A) that includes a statement of their rights as subjects and the names and phone numbers of a contact person should they have any questions. Interviews will be conducted with as much privacy as possible, preferably in the unit's 'quiet room'. Care will be taken to avoid conflict with treatments or other activities planned for the patients. During the interview, the interviewer will observe the patient carefully for signs of fatigue, and whenever the patient's condition indicates, the interviewer will stop the interview. If the patient does appear fatigued at the end of the interview, the researcher will advise the nursing staff.

Relatives

Procedures for including relatives in the study will be the same as for 'Patients'. At the beginning of each interview, an explanation of the study will be given and consent to participate in the study will be obtained. The participants will be informed that they are not required to participate in the study, that they may stop the interview at any time or refuse to answer any questions, and that whether or not they participate will have no bearing on the care that their hospitalized relative receives. The participants will be assured of anonymity, and, although some of the information they provide will be published, their name will not be associated with that publication. They will be given a copy of the informed consent form (see Appendix A) that includes a statement of their rights as subjects and the names and phone numbers of a contact person should they have any questions.

Nurses

Because of conflicting responsibilities, most of the interviews with nurses will be conducted on their own time, at the location of their choice. If interviews are conducted during the work day, the researcher will ensure that permission has been obtained from nursing administration for the nurse to be interviewed during work time. As with the patients who are subjects, at the beginning of each interview, an explanation of the study will be given and consent to participate in the study will be obtained. The participants will be informed that they are not required to participate in the study, that they may stop the interview at any time or refuse to answer any questions, and that whether or not they participate will have no bearing on their employment evaluations. The participants will be assured of anonymity, and, although some of the information they provide will be published, their name will not be associated with the publication. They will be given a copy of the informed consent form that includes a statement of their rights as subjects and the names and phone numbers of a contact person should they have any questions.

When participant observation is being conducted, the researcher will ensure that everyone present is aware of the research, has previously consented to participate in the project and is aware that data collection is proceeding at that time. If a person who has not given informed consent enters the setting, then data collection will cease, either until that person consents to participate in the study or leaves the area.

Permission will be obtained from all institutions in which data will be collected. No risks to the participants are expected. Although in previous research informants were occasionally uncomfortable discussing personal material,[14] informants found the experience therapeutic, and it enriched their daily lives. If, however, a participant becomes upset, the interviewer will remain with the participant until the crisis is over and refer the person for professional counselling. In the rare event that knowledge of inferior standards of care that endangers patient life is brought to the attention of the investigator, then the investigator will, with the knowledge of the informant, report the incident to the hospital ombudsman.

The tapes will be kept in a locked office, and all identifying information will be removed from the tapes during the transcription process. All transcripts will be coded, and the informed consent forms will be stored separately from the data.

There may be no direct benefits to participants for participating in this research; however, in previous studies, informants have reported that participating in interviews has been an enormously rewarding experience. They have stated that it was a privilege to be asked an opinion and to be listened to seriously. The real benefits of the study will be in the development of the construct of comfort and further understanding of how nurses provide comfort. Summaries of the research results will be provided to all participants, and copies of the research reports and reprints of articles will be supplied to the host institution.

I. LITERATURE CITED

1. Travelbee, J. (1976) *Intervention in Psychiatric Nursing: Process in the One-to-One Relationship*, F.A. Davis, Philadelphia.
2. Leininger, M.M. (1984) The essence of nursing and health, in *Care: The Essence of Nursing and Health*, (ed. M.M. Leininger), C.B. Slack, Thorofare, NJ, pp. 3–15.
3. Watson, J. (1978) *Nursing: The Philosophy and Science of Caring*, Little, Brown & Co., Boston.
4. Bevis, E.O. (1981) Caring: a life force, in *Caring: An Essential Human Need*, (ed. M.M. Leininger), C.B. Slack, Thorofare, NJ, pp. 49–60.
5. Gustafson, W. (1984) Motivational and historical aspects of care and nursing, in *Care: The Essence of Nursing and Health*, (ed. M.M. Leininger), C.B. Slack, Thorofare, NJ, pp. 61–74.
6. Leininger, M.M. (1981) The phenomenon of caring: importance, research questions and theoretical considerations, in *Caring: An Essential Human Need*, (ed. M.M. Leininger), C.B. Slack, Thorofare, NJ, pp. 3–15.
7. Wolf, Z.R. (1986) The caring concepts and nurse identified caring behaviors. *Topics in Clinical Nursing*, **8**(2), 84–93.
8. Leininger, M.M. (1981) Cross-cultural hypothetical functions of caring and nursing care, in *Caring: An Essential Human Need*, (ed. M.M. Leininger), C.B. Slack, Thorofare, NJ, p. 101.
9. Ray, M.A. (1984) The development of a classification system of institutional caring, in *Care: The Essence of Nursing and Health*, (ed. M.M. Leininger), C.B. Slack, Thorofare, NJ, pp. 95–112.
10. Ray, M.A. (1987) Technological caring: a new model in critical care. *Dimensions in Critical Care Nursing*, **6**(3), 166–73.
11. Dunlop, M.J. (1986) Is a science of caring possible? *Journal of Advanced Nursing*, **11**, 661–70.
12. Rieman, D.J. (1986) Noncaring and caring in the clinical setting: patients' descriptions. *Topics in Clinical Nursing*, **8**(2), 30–6.
13. Swanson-Kauffman, K. (1986) Caring in the instance of unexpected early pregnancy loss. *Topics in Clinical Nursing*, **8**(2), 37–46.
14. Morse, J.M. (1983) An ethnoscientific analysis of comfort: a preliminary investigation. *Nursing Papers/Perspectives in Nursing*, **15**(1), 6–19.
15. Brink, P. and Saunders, J. (1976) Culture shock: theoretical and applied, in *Transcultural Nursing: A Book of Readings*, (ed. P. Brink), Prentice-Hall, Englewood Cliffs, NJ, pp. 126–38.
16. Geach, B. (1987) Pain and coping. *Image: Journal of Nursing Scholarship*, **19**(1), 12–15.
17. Morse, J.M., and Morse, R.M. (1988) Evaluation of the pain experience of others: cultural variation in the perception of painful events. *Journal of Cross-Cultural Psychology*, **19**(2), 232–42.
18. Morse, J.M. (1982) 'Does it hurt?' Cultural variation in the perception of painful events, in *Transcultural Nursing*, Proceedings from the Seventh Transcultural Nursing Conference, (eds C. Uhl and J. Uhl), University of Utah and the Transcultural Nursing Society, Salt Lake City, pp. 45–53.
19. Morse, J.M., and Park, C. (1988) Hospital births and home deliveries. *Research in Nursing and Health*, **11**, 175–81.

20. Morse, J.M. and Park, C. (1988) Differences in cultural expectations of the perceived painfulness of parturition, in *Childbirth in America: Anthropological Perspectives*, (ed. K. Michaelson), Bergin and Garvey, South Hadley, MA, pp. 121–9.

21. Morse, J.M. (1989). Cultural responses to parturition: childbirth in Fiji. *Medical Anthropology*, **12**(1), 35–44.

22. Côté, J.J., Morse, J.M. and James, S.G. (1991) The pain experience of the post-operative newborn. *Journal of Advanced Nursing*, **16**, 378–87.

23. Thomas, A. and Morse, J.M. (1991) Managing urinary incontinence. *Journal of Gerontological Nursing*, **17**(6), 9–14.

24. McLeod-Engel, N. (1987) The use of TV in an extended care facility. Unpublished Master of Nursing thesis. University of Alberta, Edmonton.

25. English, J. and Morse, J.M. (1988) The 'difficult' patient: adjustment or maladjustment? *International Journal of Nursing Studies*, **25**(1), 23–39.

26. Morse, J.M., Morse, R.M. and Tylko, S. (1989) Developing a scale to identify the fall-prone patient. *Canadian Journal on Aging*, **8**(4), 366–77.

27. Morse, J.M., Black, C., Oberle, K. and Donahue, P. (1989) A prospective study to identify the fall-prone patient. *Social Sciences and Medicine*, **28**(1), 81–6.

28. Morse, J.M., Tylko, S. and Dixon, H.A. (1987) Characteristics of patients that fall. *The Gerontologist*, **27**(4), 516–22.

29. Morse, J.M. (1986) Computerized evaluation of a scale to identify the fall-prone patient. *Canadian Journal of Public Health*, **77** (suppl. I), 21–5.

30. Morse, J.M., Tylko, S.J. and Dixon, H.A. (1986) Identifying the fall-prone patient. *Nursing Research: Science for Quality Care, Proceedings of the National Nursing Research Conference*, University of Toronto, Toronto, pp. 88–92.

31. Morse, J.M., Tylko, S. and Dixon, H.A. (1985) The patient who falls ... and falls again. Defining the aged at risk. *Journal of Gerontological Nursing*, **11**(11), 15–18.

32. Morse, J.M., Prowse, M., Morrow, N. and Federspiel, G. (1985) A retrospective analysis of patient falls. *Canadian Journal of Public Health*, **76**(2), 116–18.

33. McHutchion, E. and Morse, J.M. (1989) Releasing restraints: a nursing dilemma? *Journal of Gerontological Nursing*, **15**(2), 16–21.

34. Morse, J.M., and McHutchion, E. (1991) The behavioral effects of releasing restraints. *Research in Nursing and Health*, **14**, 187–96.

35. Morse, J.M., Stedman, J. and Olmstead, D. (1985) *Development of a geriatric bed, bed alarm and chair alarm.* Proposal funded in part by the Alberta Medical Heritage Foundation and the University of Alberta Special Services Committee, Edmonton, Alberta.

36. Chassé, M.A. (1990) The experience of women undergoing hysterectomy. Unpublished Master of Nursing thesis. University of Alberta, Edmonton.

37. Johnson, J. (1988) Recovering from heart attack: experiences of men and women. Unpublished Master of Nursing thesis. University of Alberta, Edmonton.

38. Lorencz, B. (1988) Perceptions of adult chronic schizophrenics during planned discharge. Unpublished Master of Nursing thesis. University of Alberta, Edmonton.

40. Wilson, S. (1988) Living with chemotherapy: perceptions of the spouse. Unpublished Master of Nursing thesis. University of Alberta, Edmonton.

41. Morse, J.M., Young, D., Swartz, L. and McConnell, R. (1987) A Cree Indian treatment for psoriasis: a longitudinal study. *Culture*, **7**(2), 31–41.

42. Morse, J.M., McConnell, R., and Young. D. (1988) Documenting the practice of a traditional healer: methodological problems and issues, in *Health Care Issues in the Canadian North*, (ed. D. Young), Boreal Institute, Edmonton, pp. 88–94.

43. Young, D., Swartz, I., Ingram, G. and Morse J.M. (1988) The psoriasis research project: an overview, in *Health Care Issues in the Canadian North*, (ed. D. Young), Boreal Institute, Edmonton, pp. 76–87.

44. Morse, J.M. (1987) The meaning of health in an inner-city community. *Nursing Papers/Perspectives in Nursing*, **19**(2), 27–41.

45. Telford, L. (1987) Adolescent health: an emic perspective. Unpublished Master of Nursing thesis, University of Alberta, Edmonton.

46. Morse, J.M. (1984) Breast- and bottle-feeding: The effect on infant weight gain in the Fiji-Indian neonate. *Ecology of Food and Nutrition*, **15**, 109–14.

47. Morse, J.M. (1984) The cultural context of infant feeding in Fiji. *Ecology of Food and Nutrition*, **14**, 287–96.

48. Morse, J.M. and English J. (1986) The incorporation of cultural concepts in basic nursing texts. *Nursing Papers/Perspectives in Nursing*, **18**(2), 69–76.

49. Morse, J.M. (ed.) (1988) *Recent Advances in Cross-Cultural Nursing*, Churchill Livingstone, Edinburgh.

50. Morse, J.M. (1983) The inter-relationship of traditional care and clinic care for the Fiji-Indian neonate, in *Partners in Nursing Progress*, (ed. Tan Khim Han). Proceedings of the First Asian and Pacific Nurses Convention, Singapore Trained Nurses Association, Singapore, Publication No. MC(P) 101/3/83, pp. 130–32.

51. Morse, J.M. (1989) Cross-cultural nursing: a unique contribution to medical anthropology? *Medical Anthropology*, **12**, 1–5.

52. Morse, J.M. (1988) Cultural values and beliefs in health care. Paper presented at the Transcultural Health Workshop, McMaster University, Hamilton, Ontario, 27 May, 1987.

53. Morse, J.M. and Relyea, J.M. (1983) Cultural forces as a contraceptive agent: an examination of the non-technical mechanisms that influence coital activity, in *A Transcultural Nursing Challenge: From Discovery to Action*, (ed. J. Uhl). Proceedings of the Eighth Transcultural Nursing Conference, Transcultural Nursing Society, Salt Lake City, pp. 1–20.

54. Morse, J.M., Edwards J. and Kappagoda, T. (1988) The health care needs of South-east Asian refugees. *Canadian Family Practitioner*, **34**, 2351–606.

55. Morse, J.M. (1984) Health consequences of culture shock: a pilot study, in *Nursing Papers* (special supplement), *Nursing Research: A Base for Practice*, (eds M. Kravitz and J. Laurin). Proceedings of the Ninth National Conference (1983), McGill University School of Nursing, Montreal, Quebec, pp. 348–67.

56. Braxton, J., Germer, L. and Pearson (Morse), J. (1979) *Indochinese Refugees: A Guide for Sponsoring Indochinese Refugees in Utah*, Utah State Department of Social Services, Salt Lake City, (reprinted 1980, 1981).

57. Morse, J.M. and Doan, H.M. (1987) Growing up at school: adolescents response to menarche. *Journal of School Health*, **57**(9), 385–9.

58. Doan, H. and Morse, J.M. (1985) The last taboo: roadblocks for researching menarche. *Health Care for Women International*, **6**(5-6), 277–83.

59. Doan, H. and Morse, J.M. (1985) *Every Girl Learning about Menstruation*. Monograph for perimenstrual adolescents. General Publishing Co., Toronto.

60. Morse, J.M., Kieren, D. and Bottorff, J.L. (1993) The adolescent menstrual

attitude questionnaire: I scale construction. *Health Care for Women International,* **14**, 39–62.

61. Morse, J.M. (1990) 'Euch! Those are for your husband!': examination of cultural values and assumptions associated with breast-feeding. *Health Care for Women International,* **11**(2), 223–32.

62. Morse, J.M. (1982) Infant feeding in the Third World: a critique of the literature. *Advances in Nursing Science,* **5**(1), 77–88.

63. Morse, J.M. (1985) The cultural context of infant feeding in Fiji, in *Infant Feeding in Oceania,* (ed. L. Marshall), Gordon and Breach, New York, pp. 255–68.

64. Harrison, M.J., Morse, J.M., and Prowse, M. (1985) Successful breastfeeding: the mother's dilemma. *Advanced Journal of Nursing,* **10**, 261–69.

65. Morse, J.M. and Harrison, M. (1988) Patterns of mixed feeding. *Midwifery,* **4**(1), 19–23.

66. Morse, J.M., Harrison, M. and Prowse, M. (1986) Minimal breastfeeding. *Journal of Obstetric, Gynecologic, and Neonatal Nursing,* **15**(4), 333–8.

67. Williams, K.M.R. and Morse, J.M. (1989) Patterns of weaning in primiparous mothers. *MCN (The American Journal of Maternal-Child Nursing),* **14**(3), 188–92.

68. Morse, J.M., Harrison, M. and Williams, K. (1988) What determines the duration of breastfeeding?, in *Childbirth in America: Anthropological Perspectives,* (ed. K. Michaelson), Bergin and Garvey, South Hadley, MA, pp. 261–70.

69. Morse, J.M. and Harrison M. (1987) Social coercion for weaning. *Journal of Nurse-Midwifery,* **32**(4), 205–10.

70. Morse, J.M., Jehl, C. and Gamble, D. (1990) Initiating breast-feeding: a world survey of the timing of postpartum breastfeeding. *International Journal of Nursing Studies,* **3**, 303–13.

71. Greenhalgh, J. (1988) The waking behaviors of the normal neonate. Unpublished Master of Nursing thesis. University of Alberta, Edmonton.

72. Morse, J.M. (1984) *Coping with breastfeeding and work.* Proposal funded by the Alberta Foundation for Nursing Research, Edmonton.

73. Morse J.M. and Bottorff, J.L. (1988) The emotional experience of breast expression. *Journal of Nurse-Midwifery,* **33**(4), 165–70.

74. Neander, W. and Morse, J.M. (1989) The cultural context of infant feeding among the Northern Alberta Woodlands Cree. *Canadian Journal of Public Health,* **80**(3), 190–4.

75. Edwards, J. and Morse, J.M. (1989) The international growth reference: one standard for all? *Public Health Nursing,* **6**(1), 35–42.

76. Morse, J.M. and Edwards, J.E. (1987) Are people really different? Significance of the anthropomorphic racial variation. Unpublished paper, University of Alberta, Edmonton.

77. Slevin, A.P. and Harter, M.O. (1987) The teaching of caring: a survey report. *Nursing Educator,* **12**(6), 23–6.

78. Hamilton, J. (1989) Comfort and the hospitalized chronically ill. *Journal of Gerontological Nursing,* **15**(4), 28–33.

79. Flemming, C., Scanlon, C. and D'Agostina, N.S. (1987) A study of the comfort needs of patients with advanced cancer. *Cancer Nursing,* **10**(5), 237–43.

80. Leininger, M. (1981) Some philosophical, historical and taxonomic aspects of nursing caring in American culture, in *Caring: An Essential Human Need,* (ed. M.M. Leininger), C.B. Slack, Thorofare, NJ, pp. 133–44.

81. Watson, J., Buskhardt, C., Brown, L. *et al.* (1979) A model of caring: an alternative health care model for nursing practice and research, in *ANA Clinical and Scientific Sessions*, pp. 32–44.
82. Mayer, D.K. (1986) Cancer patients' and families' perceptions of nurse caring behaviors. *Topics in Clinical Nursing*, **8**(2), 63–9.
83. Field, P.A. and Morse, J.M. (1985) *Nursing Research: The Application of Qualitative Approaches*, Croom Helm, London.
84. Ray, M.A. (1987) Phenomenology: a qualitative research method. *Dimensions of Critical Care Nursing*, **6**, 69.
85. Bergum, V. (1988) *Woman to Mother: A Transformation*, Bergin & Garvey, South Hadley, MA.
86. Lear, M.W. (1980) *Heart Sounds*, Simon & Schuster, New York
87. Omery, A. (1983) Phenomenology: a method for nursing research. *Advances in Nursing Science*, **5**(2), 49–63.
88. van Manen, M. (1984) Practicing phenomenological writing. *Phenomenology + Pedagogy*, **2**(1), 35–72.
89. Tesch, R. (1987) Emerging themes: the researcher's experience. *Phenomenology + Pedagogy*, **5**(3), 230–41.
90. Ray, M.A. (1985) A philosophical method to study nursing phenomena, in *Qualitative Research Methods in Nursing*, (ed. M. Leininger), Grune & Stratton, Orlando, pp. 81–92.
91. Harris, M. (1968) *The Rise of Anthropological Theory*, Thomas Y. Cromwell, New York.
92. Morse, R.M., and Morse, J.M. (1989) *QUAL*: a mainframe program for qualitative data analysis. *Nursing Research*, **38**(3), 188–9.
93. Spradley, J. (1979) *The Ethnographic Interview*, Rinehart & Winstone, New York.
94. Evaneshko, V. and Kay, M.A. (1982) The ethnoscience technique. *Western Journal of Nursing Research*, **4**, 49–64.
95. Gerson, E.M. (1986) Computing in qualitative research: an approach to structured text. *Qualitative Sociology*, **9**(2), 204–7.
96. Prescott, P.A., Dennis, K.E. and Jacox, A.K. (1987) Clinical decision making of staff nurses. *Image*, **19**(2), 56–62.
97. Strauss, A.L., Corbin, J., Fagerhaugh, S. *et al.* (1984) *Chronic Illness and the Quality of Life*, 2nd edn, C.V. Mosby Co., St Louis.
98. Estabrooks, C. and Morse, J.M. (1992) Toward a theory of touch: the touching process and acquiring a touching style. *Journal of Advanced Nursing*, **17**, 448–56.
99. Glaser, B.G. and Strauss, A.L. (1967) *The Discovery of Grounded Theory*, Aldine Publishing, Chicago.
100. Glaser, B.G. (1978) *Theoretical Sensitivity*, The Sociology Press, San Francisco.
101. Stern, P., Allen, L. and Moxley, P. (1982) The nurse as a grounded theorist: history, process and uses. *The Review Journal of Philosophy and Social Science*, **7**(1, 2), 200–15.
102. Hutchinson, S. (1986) Grounded theory: the method, in *Nursing Research: A Qualitative Perspective*, (ed. P.L. Munhall and C.J. Oiler), Appleton-Century Crofts, Norwalk, CT, pp. 111–30.
103. Chenitz, W.C. and Swanson, J.M. (1986) *From Practice to Grounded Theory*, Addison-Wesley, Menlo Park, CA.
104. Sacks, O. (1984) *A Leg to Stand on*, Summit Books, New York.

105. Sherrard, I. (1988) Care that wasn't given. *New Zealand Nursing Journal*, **81**(1), 23.

106. Rogoff, B. (1978) Spot observation: an introduction and examination. *Institute for Comparative Human Development*, **2**(2), 21–6.

107. Morse, J.M. (1986) Qualitative and quantitative methods: issues in sampling, in *Nursing Research Methodology*, (ed. P.L. Chinn), Aspen, Rockville, MD, pp. 181–91.

108. Manning, P.K. (1982) Analytic induction, in *Qualitative Methods: Volume II of Handbook of Social Science Methods*, (eds R.B. Smith and P. Manning), Ballinger, Cambridge, MA, pp. 273–302.

109. Kvale, S. (1984) The qualitative research interview: a phenomenological and hermeneutical mode of understanding. *Journal of Phenomenological Psychology*, **14**(2), 171–96.

110. Lincoln, Y.S. and Guba, E.G. (1985) *Naturalistic Inquiry*, Sage, Beverly Hills, CA.

111. Hammersley, M. and Atkinson, P. (1983) *Ethnography: Principles and Practice*, Tavistock Publishers, London.

Appendix B
Critique of the proposal

While proposals will be either funded, invited to be revised and resubmitted or denied funding, the agency usually has the proposal evaluated by several reviewers. The input from these reviewers is then summarized, and this critique is then given back to the researcher. The critique below is the summary returned to the investigator, Janice Morse, for the proposal in Appendix A, and in this case the proposal was funded. Missing from this critique is the review of the personnel, the institution and the budget, and the priority score.

CRITIQUE

Résumé

The purpose of this study is to investigate comfort. The need for nurse scientists to explore the everyday concepts of clinical practice is evident. In terms of theory development, the proposed study can make a fine contribution. The investigator team is well qualified, has worked together in the past and is completely familiar with the proposed methodology. The aims of the study are specific and achievable with the research design outlined. The proposal lacks some procedural detail. This is an interesting, creative proposal with a research design that, in this particular study, is likely to produce data that could not be generated in any other way and that could be extraordinarily useful to nursing.

Critique

The significance of understanding essential concepts such as care and comfort for the development of nursing science cannot be underestimated. The investigator makes a good case for both the practical and theoretical significance of the proposed study and its potential contribution to nursing theory. The specific aims of the research — to delineate the construct of comfort; to identify the components of comfort; to identify the process of comfort — are clearly stated and appropriate. The background and significance section of the proposal explicates the notion of comfort and distinguishes it from caring in a major theoretical shift. The investigator argues cogently that this offers several advantages, including greater clinical relevance (since the focus will be the patient rather than the nurse) and greater potential for measurability. Although the assumption of an illness–health continuum is debatable, this seems a relatively minor point and does not influence the conceptual distinction between comfort and care. The investigators familiarity with the literature on caring is evident, and her alternative of comfort is based on a thoughtful and creative understanding of that literature. For several years, the investigator and her colleagues have conducted studies to further delineate the components and meaning of comfort in a broad variety of contexts, either by focusing directly on comfort or on its opposites, distress and suffering. The proposed study would depart from previous work in its concentration on ill persons; specifically, hospitalized patients across the life span, rather than on healthy subjects. The investigator is convincing in her defence of phenomenology and an inductive approach for the development of nursing theory in this particular study. Her designation of human responses which nurses must address is a useful way of organizing her explication of the concept of comfort from her previous work.

The phenomenological approach is well suited to the first study, and the investigator is obviously knowledgeable about the phenomenology method and its limitations. Her examples of broad and encouraging questions, such as, 'Tell me about your illness from the beginning', are appropriate, and she provides useful examples of the technique. In Study II, the Components of Comfort, the investigator shifts to the notion of comfort as action. In this component, she uses an ethnoscience approach in which one creates a taxonomy by identifying from interview data, contrasting and comparable things. The assumptions on which this technique is based, that informants' 'models' are consistent and shared through culture (and therefore one interview can begin where another left off rather than using the same questions), is not held by all anthropologists and probably needs a more convincing justification. It also presumes that the object of the research, in this case comfort, is at the level of consciousness so that it can be retrieved on interview from the informant. Direct observations of non-verbal behaviour, which could be very helpful, particularly with hospitalized patients potentially in crisis, are not included in the method. The investigator has outlined standard procedures for ethnoscience, however, and is qualified to carry it out. More detail regarding why triadic and dyadic card sorts are essential to the development of a taxonomy would be helpful. The investigator describes a computer technique that can facilitate the content analysis after coding which she developed. This is an important breakthrough in research methodology. Study III, the Explication of the Process of Comforting, shifts to comfort as a process. The investigator identifies many of the problems associated with nursing procedures that, because of their non-technical nature, are devalued in a patient care setting. Using a grounded theory approach, the investigator again will select an initial purposeful sample, including 25 practising nurses, 10 patients who are also nurses and 10 patient relatives who are also nurses. Importantly, this component also included direct observation. The management of data is carefully explained and demonstrates the investigators familiarity with the method.

Reliability and validity are addressed through the selection of purposeful samples, the quality of the informant, and the interaction between the informant and the interviewer. The potential for interviewer bias is addressed through 'bracketing' and subsequent analysis of the transcripts. Essentially, bias is addressed by accounting for it rather than removing it. According to the protocol, all interviews will be checked for accuracy and omissions, but the investigator does not say by whom. Self-selection bias, as a limitation, could have been more adequately addressed. The data analysis has been discussed throughout the methods section, and the discussion is adequate.

Glossary

Coding
The process of identifying persistent words, phrases, themes or concepts within the data so that the underlying patterns can be identified and analysed.

Common sense knowledge
Common sense knowledge has been described as the socially sanctioned facets of life in society that any bonafide member of the society knows and which are necessary for individuals to have in order to function in that society. The knowledge may be implicit and unconscious, to be recognized only when the norms of behaviour are violated (for example unspoken rules relating to personal space).

Concept
A phenomenon which has been identified by common recognition or by formal definition.

Conceptual framework
A theoretical model developed to show relationships between constructs. It is often used in qualitative research for the identification of variables.

Construct
A term comprising several concepts which is, therefore, more encompassing and more abstract than a single concept.

Deduction
The process of inferring future outcome from previous research or prior theoretical speculation.

Deductive theory
Variables, concepts, constructs and hypotheses are derived from previous research and relationships are tested during the research process. Theory is used to guide data collection and analysis.

Emic
The study and analysis of a setting or behaviour interpreted from the author's perspective. Thus, cultural explanations and patterns are inductively 'discovered' within the cultural context rather than analysed from the researcher's perspective or on a prior framework or theory.

Etic
The study and analysis of behaviour interpreted from the perspective of the observer. Etic analysis of events and patterns permits cross-cultural generalizations to be made.

Generalizability
Generalizability is the extent to which the findings of the research may be applied to other situations or settings.

Grounded theory
A primarily inductive approach to theory development in which emerging hypotheses are tested deductively and subsequent theory and data collection modified until the optimal fit between the data and theory has been obtained.

Hypothesis
A proposition or a predicted relationship between variables.

Inductive theory
Variables, concepts, constructs and hypotheses are derived from relationships observed during the process of coding the data. Thus, theory is constructed to explain the observed relationships as they emerge from the data.

Informants
Members of the social or cultural group in the research context who provide information and assistance with the interpretation of the setting. A key informant is the informant from whom the majority of information is obtained. Secondary informants are used by the researcher to confirm or refute the information (provided by the key informant), to widen the database as theory is developed or to search for negative cases.

Lexeme
A local name, or a label or slang term used to describe or refer to characteristics of a person, object, place or thing.

Life-world phenomena
The life-world is the world of everyday life, that is the total sphere of experiences of an individual within the context of the objects, persons and events encountered in everyday life.

Meaning
Meaning is the interpretation that informants place on the rules, issues and behaviour of the culture. The researcher must determine how the informant classifies information. The role of the researcher is to explain the meaning of the behaviour of a particular society, that is to make the implicit knowledge explicit. The interpretation of the meaning is the informant's privilege, while the mode of explanation is the researcher's.

Paradigm
A collection of logically connected concepts and propositions that provides a theoretical perspective or orientation that frequently guides research approaches towards a topic.

Participant
An individual who provides the researcher with information relevant to the study or who consents to be observed during the course of the research. Informants are also participants and the two terms may be used interchangeably. A participant is a subject in the quantitative study.

Phenomenology
Phenomenology is a philosophy and a research approach that focuses on the meaning of the 'lived experience'. The intention is to examine and describe phenomena as they appear in the lived experience of the individual. Thus, human experience is inductively derived and described with the purpose of discovering the essence of meaning.

Qualitative methods
Inductive, holistic, emic, subjective and process-oriented research methods used to understand, interpret, describe and develop theory pertaining to a phenomenon or a setting.

Quantitative methods
Positivistic, deductive, particularistic, objective research methods primarily designed to test hypotheses or establish relationships.

Reliability
The measure of the extent to which random variation may have influenced stability and consistency of the results.

Respondent
A person who voluntarily consents to complete a questionnaire or survey.

Subject
A participant in a research project usually used by the researcher to test hypotheses.

Taxonomy
A classification system which organizes components into sub-categories (or sub-segregates) according to common characteristics.

Theory
The researcher's perception of reality in which concepts are identified, relationships are proposed and predictions are made or results prescribed.

Thick description
Thick description presents more than superficial commentary on the ongoing activities. Thick description includes details of the affects, relationships, contexts, backgrounds, and interprets the tones of the voices, the feelings and meaning of the situation.

Triangulation
The use of two or more methods to examine the same phenomenon simultaneously or sequentially.

Understanding
Understanding is the discovery of the ways in which a culture accomplishes its human ends: why the approach works for the specific culture; and under what circumstances an approach works to achieve the desired ends. Understanding is the process of discovering the insider's perspective on the situation.

Validity
In qualitative research, validity refers to the extent to which the research findings represent reality.

Variables
These are the measurable characteristics of a concept and consist of logical groups of attributes.

Author Index

Subject Index